WP WELL BEING SERIES

asthma

Less Attacks, No Attacks

Marian Slee

Published by
Wilkinson Publishing Pty Ltd
ACN 006 042 173
Level 4, 2 Collins Street, Melbourne, Vic 3000
Tel: 03 9654 5446 www.wilkinsonpublishing.com.au

International distribution by Pineapple Media Ltd
(www.pineapple-media.com)
Copyright © 2014 Marian Slee

National Library of Australia Cataloguing-in-Publication entry:

Author: Slee, Marian, author.

Title: Asthma : less attacks, no attacks / Marian Slee.

ISBN: 9781922178695 (paperback)

Series: WP well being series.

Subjects: Asthma.
               Asthma--Alternative treatment.
               Vitamin therapy.

Dewey Number: 616.23806

Photos and illustrations by agreement with international agencies,
photographers and illustrators from iStockphoto.

Design: Jo Hunt
Printed in China

About the author

Marian grew up in the town of Biloela, Queensland, Australia. She and husband Jim, lived in Brisbane for 43 years and have six children. She now resides in Newcastle, New South Wales.

At age 27, Marian developed asthma and suffered regularly for eight years. In 1980, she accidentally stumbled across the amazing effects of vitamins A and E on her asthma. After successfully treating herself, she felt compelled to spread the message to others. Letters to the Editor, Talk Back Radio and magazine articles were some of her methods.

In 1996, she wrote and had published her first book, *Give Asthma the Big A*. It became a best seller in Australia.

She attempted to influence health professionals, and although some surprised her by their acceptance, most were negative. The feedback from followers of this vitamin approach however, has always been positive, and is typified by this response from the mother of an asthmatic child:

'If they invented a drug as good as this, it would be hailed a wonder drug.'

Acknowledgements

I wish to express my sincere gratitude to all who have generously contributed their own, or their children's, asthma experiences. Their stories have inspired me to continue striving to publicise the vitamin approach to asthma.

Thank you again to Betty and Beverley who helped and encouraged me in the writing of my earlier edition.

And finally, I extend my love and appreciation to my family – in particular those who assisted with the final production of this book.

Contents

Before we start: Some Asthma Facts and Findings

By Sam Wilkinson

Introduction

With no cure discovered yet, there are millions around the world who are managing their asthma. For many, every day is a struggle to stay on top of their symptoms and avoid anything that can trigger them. I'm one of them. I've been an asthmatic all my life.

When I was very little I used to get serious asthma attacks, some which required hospitalization (although they were never for too long, usually a day at most). I have since been quite lucky. By my teenage years, my asthma was relatively under control. I stopped having the severe asthma attacks, and my breathing was what I considered to be 'normal'. As teenagers tend to do however, I got a bit careless with keeping it under control, and so went off any asthma medication that I had been taking when I was younger. That was fine until I reached my mid-20s and I found the shortness of breath beginning to return. I enjoy running as a form of keeping fit, so it became a real problem for me. Nowadays I try to pay closer attention to my treatment, and have some inhalers to help me through my day. However I am always looking at different suggestions for making things a bit better.

Asthma: Less Attacks, No Attacks explores one way to make things better: the effect that vitamins, especially vitamin A, can have in easing the wheezing and shortness of breath. Like myself, author Marian Slee, is an asthmatic. Her symptoms developed later in life compared to mine, and were more severe and difficult to treat. After years of frustration at being unable to control her asthma with the more traditional types of treatment, Marian began to look for what else may work for her.

This book is the culmination of that search, with Marian now having enjoyed more than three decades of being virtually asthma-free. Before we take a look at Marian's approach however, it's timely that we learn a bit about asthma, and explore some of the other methods to treat it. Not everyone responds to particular types of treatment the same way, so we encourage readers to look at these approaches with an open mind. And above all else, we urge readers to consult their doctors on their plans for managing their asthma symptoms.

Some Numbers

Asthma is widespread. According to the World Health Organisation around 235 million people worldwide are asthmatic. Australia has as many as 2 million people with asthma symptoms to some degree. In the United Kingdom, the figure is around 5.4 million people. And in the United States, there are an estimated 25 million asthmatics. Millions more will have asthma over the next few decades, potentially as many as 100 million extra people by 2025.

Among adults, women are more likely to have asthma than men. However that is reversed in the younger age groups, with more boys under the age of 14 reported to have asthma than girls. This younger group is also more likely to require hospital treatment for their asthma symptoms, although deaths are more likely to occur amongst severe asthma-sufferers aged 65 or older. With all that being said, from 1989 to 2006, there has been an almost 70 per cent decrease in mortality rates associated with asthma.

The cost of treating asthma symptoms is among the largest contributors to healthcare expenses in many countries. In Australia, health care spending in 2004 and 2005 due to asthma came in at $606 million, or 1.2% of the total healthcare cost. In the UK, the NHS spends around a billion dollars a year treating and caring for asthmatics. And in the United States, a massive $56 billion was spent in 2007 treating asthma.

Perhaps the most concerning statistics surround peoples' attitudes to asthma. In Australia, just over a fifth of asthmatics have a written Asthma Action Plan. This is a document created with the help of a doctor that outlines what a person should do to manage their asthma on a daily basis, and what steps to take when their symptoms become more severe. Up to 90% of people with asthma inhalers do not use the proper types, or administer them the correct way. Common issues are people relying too heavily on reliever medication to control their symptoms on a daily basis, or people not using the best inhaling technique to properly receive a dose. And perhaps most concerning of all, it is estimated that as many as half of people over the age of 55 with asthma, do not actually know they have it, as they have never been properly diagnosed.

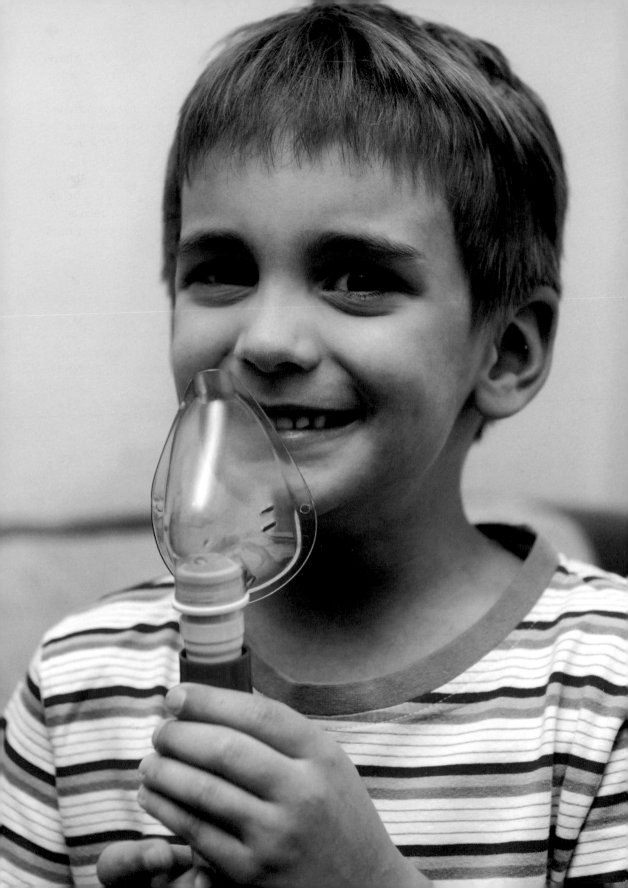

Our knowledge of Asthma over the Centuries

Asthma has been around for thousands of years. Among the earliest humans it is likely that there were some who had breathing problems associated with what we in modern times would refer to as 'asthma'.

As far as recorded history goes, there are mentions of asthma-like symptoms as far back as 2600 BCE. A disorder characterised by 'noisy breathing' was found in China, and is likely the earliest written reference to respiratory distress. The Babylonian 'Code of Hummarabi' (1792-1750 BC) recorded symptoms of breathlessness, "If a man's lungs pant with his work". Hippocrates (circa. 400 BC) identified the relationship between the environment and respiratory disease by correlating climate and location with illness. Indeed, the very name 'asthma' is a Greek word, derived from aazein, meaning to pant or exhale with an open mouth.

Moving slightly closer to today and a 17th Century Belgian physician by the name of Jean Baptiste Van Helmont was among the first to declare that asthma symptoms originated in the pipes of the lungs.

A contemporary of his, Bernadino Ramazzini (sometimes referred to as 'the father of sports medicine') was the first to detect a link between asthma and organic dust. He also recognised the symptoms for exercise-induced asthma.

On top of our understanding of what exactly asthma is, and what causes it, treatments also certainly managed to evolve over the centuries. The Jewish Talmud of 200 to 500 AD counselled drinking 'hitith', a resin from the carrot family, as a form of asthma therapy. The South American Incas treated asthma with a cocaine-like dried leaf.

Progressing into the 20th Century, the first reference made to epiphrine for the treatment of asthma came in 1905. The first use of oral cortisteroids came in the 1950s, while inhaled cortisteroids and selective short-acting beta agonist started to be used widely from the 1960s. Doctors and medical researchers have since found that inhaled bronchodilator medications aren't as likely to stimulate the heart and are available in both short and long-acting forms.

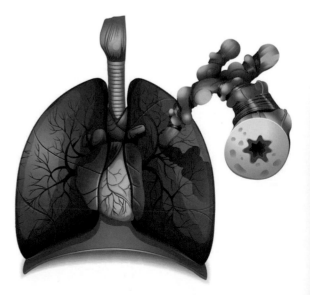

Common Ways to Treat Asthma in the 21st Century

The past couple of decades have brought us much greater understanding of asthma, although there is still no cure unfortunately. However, as many people who have had asthma can attest, the symptoms can come and go as people age. Sometimes children grow out of their symptoms, or many years of regular treatment with anti-inflammatory medication may make it disappear. On the flip side however, the symptoms can just as easily return later on in life. Many people may think of themselves as 'cured' of asthma only to find themselves once again experiencing those same symptoms.

Dealing with asthma symptoms is a must. It is not something that can simply be left alone in the hope that things will improve by themselves. There is always a risk that untreated symptoms will deteriorate over time. Poorly treated asthma gets worse with age, and the lungs of people with untreated asthma function less well than those of individuals who do not have asthma. Most doctors will advise patients to take regular, preventative asthma treatment to stop the symptoms from getting worse, and help preserve proper lung function.

The sort of treatment for asthma that is commonly recommended has changed markedly over the past 25 years. In the early 1990s, the use of nebulizers were far more commonplace. The bulky devices contained a breathing mask, which an asthma-patient would hold or attach to their mouth and inhale the medicine pumped through as a type of mist. It typically took around 5 minutes for the proper dosage to be administered. A long time for many. Since then however, the use nebulizer treatments has decreased, as the use of inhaled anti-inflammatory agents has increased.

There are different types of inhaled anti-inflammatory agents an asthma-patient can use, depending on their symptoms and the severity of their asthma overall. Doctors typically prescribe patients some form of 'preventer' medication. This medication is typically dispensed from an inhaler, and is designed to make the airways less sensitive, reduce any redness and swelling, and help to dry up mucus. Asthma patients are advised to take their preventer medication every day, once or twice, to keep their symptoms under control. They are not designed to work straight away, and should not be relied on to

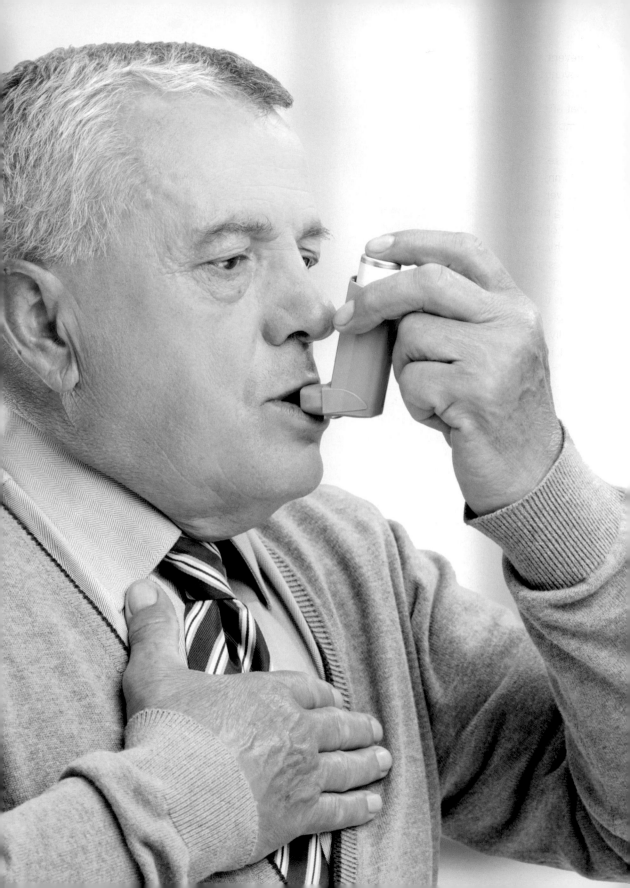

prevent an imminent asthma attack. Instead, preventer medications work to build up a person's tolerance to asthma symptoms so that after typically three to four weeks, those symptoms are much more under control.

A more immediate form of inhaled anti-inflammatory treatment comes by way of 'reliever' medication. These are the faster-acting medications, designed to give quick relief of asthma symptoms (such as wheezing, coughing and shortness of breath). They are designed to relax the muscles that are starting to constrict the airways, which in turn opens up the airways and allows for more complete breathing. Asthma patients are usually advised to have reliever medication on hand, but are only meant to take them when their symptoms flare up for immediate relief. They are not meant to be used regularly, in the place of preventer medication. A common mistake many asthmatics make is to rely solely on their reliever medication, because they think their asthma is not so severe as to require more frequent medication. They take an inhaled dose just for when any symptoms develop, instead of using preventer medication as a long term strategy to control their asthma. Asthma Australia warns that this can actually increase the long-term likelihood of the more severe asthma symptoms developing. Anyone using just a reliever medication in that fashion is strongly advised to speak to a doctor about their asthma-prevention strategies.

There are also 'symptom controllers', which act as longer-acting relievers and help to relax the muscles around the airways. As opposed to reliever medication, which typically last around 4 hours, symptom controllers will work for around 12 hours, and patients are advised to use them twice daily to relieve any severe asthma symptoms. These are prescribed for people with asthma who are already taking their regular inhaled medication, but still have persistent asthma symptoms that need addressing.

As one of the world's most prevalent diseases, there is always a considerable amount of research going into finding new ways to treat asthma. Again as previously mentioned, there is no cure, but doctors, medical researchers and scientists around the world are exploring ways to potentially find a cure, or at the very least find even better ways to reduce the symptoms of those who suffer the worst.

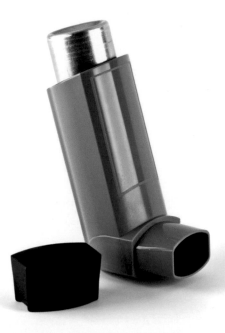

Research and Future Developments in Asthma Treatment

There has been a lot of research into the association between viral infections and asthma, especially in children who have allergic tendencies. It's well understood that the common cold can act as a trigger for severe asthma symptoms, even in people whose asthma is usually well controlled. Researchers in the United States and Australia have suggested that the severity of the illness, the type of virus and a person's allergic tendencies can all play a role in the development of persistent wheezing symptoms and asthma. Further studies into this relationship may provide new opportunities for treatment, relating to the progression from early viral infections to asthma.

Doctors are also working on ways to more accurately assess the level of inflammation in a person's lungs. There is no direct link between the severity of asthma symptoms and lung inflammation. This can make it hard for doctors to be sure that any medication, such as inhaled cortisteroids, works as intended to control that lung inflammation. One significant development over the past decade has been measuring the amount of nitric oxide in a person's inhaled breath. Nitric oxide is normally in many systems of the body and plays a vital role in inflammation. The levels can be used to indicate whether medication is likely to be effective. Doctors can measure a patient's exhaled Nitric Oxide levels to help them decide what treatments and medication doses may be necessary at all stages of treating the asthma and its symptoms.

One particular type of treatment is showing a lot of promise, but it is not for everyone. Bronchial thermoplasty is a new type of surgery. Its aim is to reduce the asthma symptoms by reducing the amount of muscle surrounding the airways in the lungs. How this is achieved is by inserting a long, flexible tube through the nose and down the into the lungs until it reaches the airways. Radio waves heat up the wires, which in turn heats the airway in a controlled manner, causing some of the muscle surrounding the airways to break up. This can help an asthmatic as those muscles tend to be thicker than in people who don't show any symptoms. However the procedure is still relatively new, and there are a limited number of places that offer it. In the United States, it can be extremely expensive and many health insurers won't cover it, as they see it as an experimental treatment. In the United Kingdom and Australia, it is only recommended for people who are aged 18 or older, and have moderate to severe asthma.

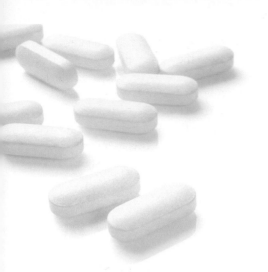

Even so, for those eligible asthmatics who have undergone the procedure there has been some success. Patients with severe asthma, which was not well controlled with the more traditional medical therapy, and who underwent this procedure in clinical trials subsequently had fewer symptoms, enjoyed a better quality of life, and needed less intensive health care (for example, emergency room visits) than patients who did not undergo the procedure.

There have been some studies that suggested a link between taking paracetamol and asthma. However at this stage the evidence is not conclusive one way or another, and more specific trials would be needed to determine if there is any causal link. So until this is known, paracetamol remains the preferred drug for pain relief and fever in children, especially as other drugs such as ibuprofen can trigger the symptoms in a small percentage of asthmatics.

Studies have also been run into how best to manage out-of-control asthma symptoms in pregnant women. Researchers at Monash University in Australia found many pregnant asthmatics would stop taking their medication out of fear for harming their baby. This actually created a far worse risk, with poorly controlled asthma sometimes leading to premature birth, low birth weight and pre-eclampsia. As many as 70 per cent of pregnant asthmatics were completely unaware of these risks. Reviews of medication have found no evidence to support this theory that they cause harm to the child. University researchers set up an intervention program for 60 women in local hospitals, and found that monthly monitoring of the asthma symptoms led to a significant reduction in out of control asthma, and successfully overcame barriers to asthma control during the pregnancy.

One of the big issues asthmatics face is how many times throughout the day they need to use their medication. While many people are able to remember the proper times, morning and night, to administer their dose, there are always plenty of people who don't.

In Britain, the first once-a-day inhaler has been introduced for prescription to adults and adolescents over the age of 12. The new drug – Relvar Ellipta – combines the daily dose of steroids to reduce the inflammation, with a new type of long acting beta2 agonist, which can dilate the airways. This new treatment provided 24 hour help for asthmatics, as opposed to the twice-a-day medication that many people either forget to use or use incorrectly.

And finally, a study that could change the way asthma symptoms are prevented has been conducted by the University of Texas Medical Branch. The study involved more than 300 adults with mild to moderate asthma, and divided them into three groups. One group received an adjusted dose of steroids and took them as usual, another group had the steroid levels adjusted after taking sophisticated asthma breath tests, and a third group used inhalers only when their symptoms flared up. Researchers found that the latter group did just as well as the first two groups, despite using just half the amount of medication. Potentially, these findings could be applied to wider asthmatic populations and significantly reduce their costs of acquiring medication.

Others Ways to Treat Asthma: Alternative Medicine and Diet

There are a variety of alternative treatments open to asthma patients, each with varying degrees of effectiveness. Much of the time, this effectiveness depends entirely on the individual and what works for them.

One idea is to employ various breathing exercises. Different techniques, used for varying lengths of time, have had some impact if they focus on awareness of breathing and control of breathing. For example, one breathing exercise, called 'buteyko breathing' focuses on breathing through the nose, taking smaller, slower breaths and avoiding deep breaths. However there isn't much evidence showing any improvement in the underlying lung inflammation or function, nor is there any change in carbon dioxide levels.

Many people feel that employing forms of relaxation therapy can have a positive effect on their breathing and state of mind. Massage, or any treatment involving manipulating the body with pressure, mainly on the soft tissue, or muscular parts of the body, can be helpful in lowering a person's stress levels. High stress is known to be a common trigger for asthma symptoms to occur.

Herbal medicine is another popular method of reducing asthma symptoms. The idea being to use treatments made from plants and plant extracts. This is one of the oldest forms of medicine used throughout the world. There is some evidence that various herbs can improve asthma symptoms, however the benefits are generally less than what would be gained from even the smallest dose of an inhaled cortisteroid preventer medication. Another significant problem is the lack of standardisation of contents and dosage, as well as the risk of side effects occurring.

Exercise seems like a contradictory method to lessen the asthma symptoms. After all, it's common for many people to trigger their shortness of breath and other asthma symptoms by simply undertaking exercise. As many as 90 per cent of asthmatics find that exercise, especially when performed in cold,

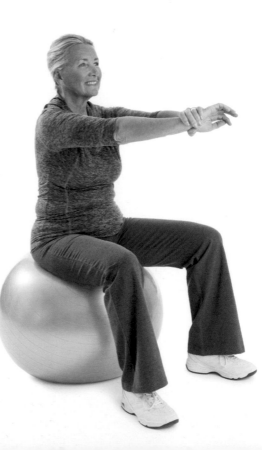

dry air is a trigger for their symptoms. Even so, the benefits of cardiovascular exercise are hugely important. With proper medication and vigilant monitoring of their symptoms, asthmatics should endeavour to work on their weight and overall fitness. Doctors especially encourage children who have asthma to remain active to strengthen their lung capacity as they grow.

There are also some links between what asthmatics eat and the extent to which their symptoms manifest. One study of adult asthmatics has found that as many as 79 per cent of respondents who had tried a restricted diet of some fashion did report improvement in their asthma symptoms. Like other forms of alternative treatment however, each person will respond differently to different foods. What may make one person's asthma symptoms worse, or better for that matter, may make no noticeable difference to another person.

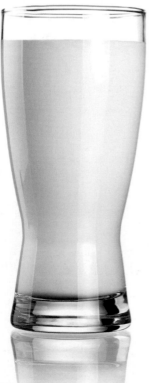

Dairy tends to have a bad reputation when it comes to asthma symptoms. It's often cited as one food group that plays a major role in exacerbating asthma symptoms. Products such as milk, cheese or yoghurt have a texture and consistency that can increase the production of mucus and congest the airways. This makes it more difficult to breathe freely. However there is no concrete, scientific evidence to support this way of thinking. In fact, there is research to suggest that dairy may actually help to protect children in particular. Nutritionists recommend dairy foods as part of a healthy, balanced diet for most people with asthma, because of the unique combination of at least 10 essential nutrients.

Different people will blame different food products in the belief that they are making their asthma symptoms worse. Common culprits are foods that can cause allergies in some people, such as eggs and peanuts, as they can tighten the airways and create all sorts of problems. Salt can cause inflammation, which is a hallmark feature of asthma, and tighten the airways and lead to fluid retention.

On the other hand, there is a whole range of food products that gets commonly cited as being more beneficial and helping to improve an asthmatic's symptoms. Studies have shown that people who have reported eating 2 to 5 apples a week had a 32 per cent lower risk of asthma. Carrots contain beta-carotine, which is connected to vitamin A in the body and may reduce the incidence of exercise induced asthma. Coffee is thought to modestly improve airway function for as long as four hours after it is consumed. And Flax Seeds are high in Omega 3 fatty acids, as well as magnesium. There is research which suggests that Omega 3's have a beneficial effect on asthma, although that research is preliminary.

Some studies have also been conducted into the effects of fibre – in particular, eating more fruit and vegetables. The University of Lausanne in Switzerland conducted tests on mice and found that those given high fibre diets were less likely to suffer serious respiratory symptoms such as the inflammation of the lungs and airways. Extra soluble fibre, commonly found in fruit and vegetables, was converted into short chain fatty acids, a type of fat which acts a signal to make the immune system more resistant to irritation. The researchers have suggested a fatty acid supplement pill could be used to treat asthma, if dietary changes cannot be made. They also argued that the boom in processed food consumption in the western world over the past 40 years is a possible explanation for why asthma rates increased over the 1980s and 90s in particular.

Sam Wilkinson is a writer /editor living in Melbourne, Australia. He has had asthma from a young age.

Dear Readers,

It's wonderful to be able to report that at 71 years of age, I am still asthma free. This amazing vitamin treatment has allowed me to enjoy over thirty years of good health. Hundreds of others have also experienced this. Admittedly, there is still the occasional cold and flu, but asthma does not develop.

Since the previous edition seven years ago, life has been very eventful. Jim and I enjoyed some exciting overseas trips and cruises. There were also some extremely traumatizing events, but apart from one year when I neglected to take vitamin C and consequently suffered repeated chest infections, the vitamins have kept me healthy.

Since that year of illness, I've never missed a daily dose of vitamin C, and it has paid off beautifully.

To all new readers of my book, I'm sure when you know my story and examine the evidence within, you will feel a renewed optimism towards your illness.

My wish for you, therefore, is vibrant good health and happiness,

Marian

Introduction

The continuing high incidence of asthma is the catalyst for this book. In it, I describe my personal discovery of a simple but controversial management and prevention programme for this illness.

News of untimely asthma deaths motivated me to share what I've learnt from more than twenty years of experimentation and research. Watching fellow sufferers enduring the side effects of drugs because no alternative treatment is countenanced distressed me greatly.

Now, in the new millennium, the buzz words, 'What works, is peer to peer,' reflect the growing recognition that people in the same situation, can help each other immensely. Why should only medical professionals write about asthma? Asthmatics are experts also. We own the illness and we alone know how it feels. Medical practitioners cannot experience our distress or the side effects of the medications they prescribe – unless they themselves are asthmatic.

When an authority extols the virtues of drug therapy, while at the same time rejecting any possibility of an effective alternative, I see **red**.

I am confident the message within this book will be good news for asthmatics everywhere. This treatment, when fully accepted and followed, has in my experience, seldom been known to fail.

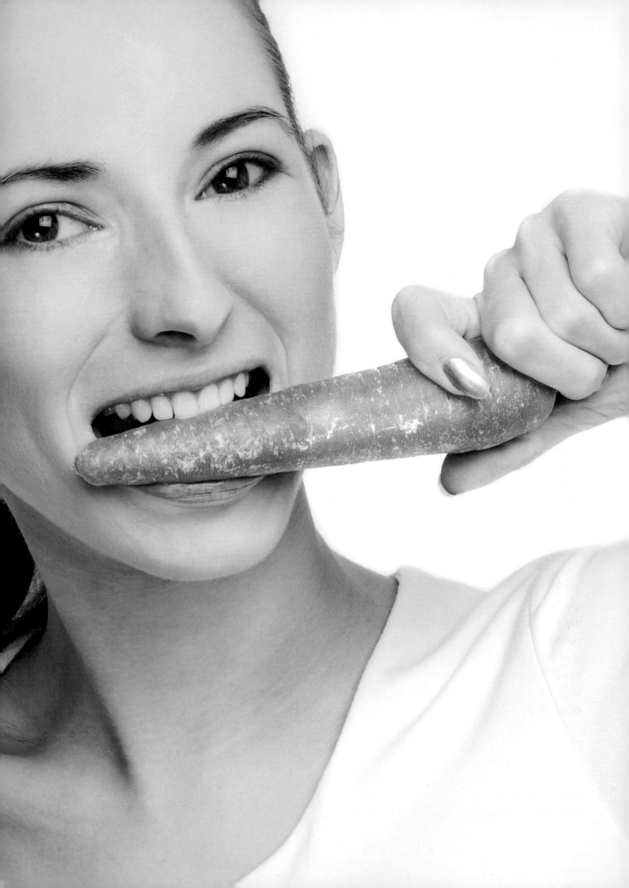

What's the problem with vitamin A?

Why all the fuss about vitamin A? Why is this vitamin constantly targeted and demonised?

Obviously the scientists who named the vitamins, didn't consider it a problem. They gave it top billing, where it has remained to this day. They believed any nutrient as hard-working as vitamin A: responsible for good eyesight, the health of linings of the respiratory and gastrointestinal tracts, the maintenance of adrenal glands and catalyst of their hormones, deserved a very important position. Naming it Vitamin A undoubtedly made good sense to them.

As it is responsible for so many activities in the body, it also follows that a shortage can have catastrophic effects. Throughout my 33 years using this vitamin, I've never suffered one side effect, yet I've been warned repeatedly of dire consequences. Strangely, none of those issuing warnings has shown the slightest interest in the fact that I've been free of asthma for 33 years!

'You will damage your liver!' was the first constant cry. 'Don't you know this vitamin accumulates?' Well, I recently undertook a liver function test with one of the leading pathologists in Queensland, and the results came back 'normal'. My kidney test was also 'normal'. And this after moderate to high doses the entire time.

'Vitamin A causes birth defects!' was another warning. For the past ten years, the labels on most vitamin A capsules claimed taking any more than 2,500 i.u. (international unit) per day could cause birth defects. What an absurd statement? Thank goodness things have improved a little as the label on my latest bottle says 'When taken in excess of 8,000 i.u. vitamin A can cause birth defects.' This is still outrageous but slightly more acceptable. While pregnant with twins, I took the occasional 5,000 i.u. vitamin A capsule, and those girls were amazingly healthy children.

The latest scare-tactic comes from Denmark. On a recent *Catalyst* programme, Danish researchers claimed vitamin A causes osteoporosis. Steroids have been implicated in the development of osteoporosis, but this was the first I'd heard of an association with vitamin A.

I underwent a bone density test after hearing this, and was told I had the bones of a 56 year old – I was 58 at the time.

It was interesting to note a scientist interviewed on *Catalyst* said he held grave doubts about the Danish research. So all the dire consequences of vitamin A have not eventuated. Would they occur in anyone, I wonder? If I haven't experienced them, who would? Many have developed a fear of vitamin A, but what is the alternative? Does anyone believe steroids could be taken for 33 years without serious side effects?

Many vitamin A warnings are not against high doses, mind you, just any vitamin A at all! And harping about overdosing to asthmatics actually deficient in vitamin A is absurd. I will never be afraid of this vitamin. It has given me so many healthy years. I wonder if the scare-mongers know of Lady Cilento's assertion that vitamin A overdose symptoms are completely **reversible** upon cessation of the vitamin.

This uproar could be understandable if the orthodox approach to asthma was a raging success but every asthmatic I've spoken with has been on two or more types of medication and **still** experiencing asthma symptoms. Surely the fact they ring me demonstrates their dissatisfaction.

Nurses trained in the 1950s say they were taught 'alternative medicine is pure quackery and no notice must be taken of it whatsoever'. If alternative medicine is quackery, does this mean the champion of the vitamin cause, Dr Linus Pauling, the only person to win two Nobel Prizes and acclaimed the world's greatest chemist, is a quack?

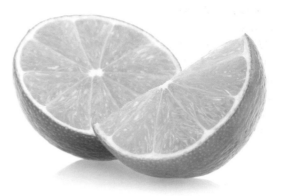

Whenever a cure from vitamins is reported the usual response is, 'Oh, that's just the placebo effect.' Anyone would think it an obscenity to claim vitamins could alleviate so serious a disease as asthma.

Captain Cook must have shocked many when he stated, to prevent scurvy, he was loading limes and pickled vegetables onto his ship. Lady Cilento wrote scurvy was one of the most feared killer diseases of all time, claiming more victims than the plague.

Obtaining scientific evidence on vitamins is very difficult and almost a lost cause. Even Dr Pauling in 1989 said because of lack of funds, he was experiencing severe difficulties continuing with his experiments. No one can claim ownership of a vitamin, so there is little incentive to finance research. A patent can be taken out on a drug, but a vitamin is simply an organic compound.

Which makes one wonder why almost ten years ago, we were hearing of research portraying a negative effect from taking vitamin A.

The Office of Dietary Supplements, National Institutes of Health, Maryland, USA, distributes excellent information on vitamin A but also includes some negative and unbelievable studies. Their 2005 fact sheet begins by detailing the wonderful functions vitamin A performs in the body, and continues, 'There is increased interest in sub clinical forms of vitamin A deficiency, described as low storage levels of vitamin A that do not cause overt deficiency symptoms. This mild degree of vitamin A deficiency may increase children's risk of developing respiratory and diarrheal infections, decrease growth rate, slow bone development and decrease likelihood of survival from serious illness.'

Another section states, 'Surveys suggest an association between diets rich in beta-carotene and vitamin A, and a lower risk of many types of cancer'. This is fantastic. However, it finishes by describing two recent studies: The first found that 'lung cancer among smokers was 18% higher in those who took beta-carotene supplements', than those who took a placebo. The second, (a lung cancer chemo prevention study) claims subjects who were given '30mg beta-carotene and 25,000 i.u. of vitamin A per day, had a 46% higher risk of dying from lung cancer than those who took a placebo.'

These results are incredible and I can't believe anyone could take them seriously. Still, they made headlines around the world. However the research was later discredited. Dr Isabelle Bairati from Quebec Research Centre, advised in 2008 that she got it wrong. After re-examining the data, it was found the only patients who saw their cancer return were smokers who refused to give up their habit while undergoing radiation and chemotherapy (Source: International Journal of Cancer, 2008; 122: 1679-83).

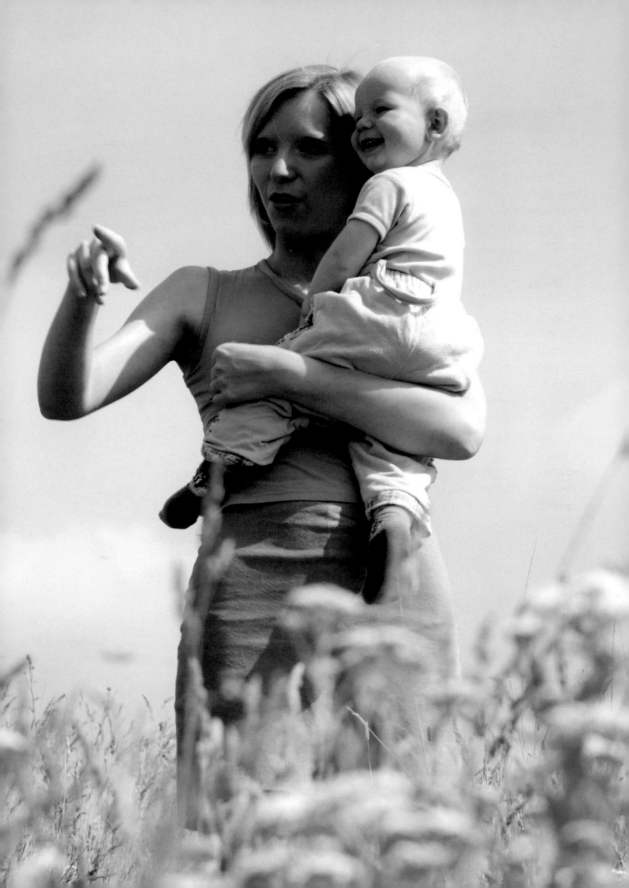

Early days

Asthma – I had it, now I don't.

During my late twenties and thirties, I dreaded every respiratory infection and change in the season. Now I live as though asthma was never a part of my life. Allow me to tell you my story.

Asthma became a reality for me in the winter of 1969. I was twenty-seven, married and the mother of three small boys. Earlier that year we were transferred to Brisbane and in August I contracted Hong Kong 'Flu. Each time I attempted to stand, severe infection and high temperatures made me faint and fall. I was worried.

How could I feed my three-month-old son if I couldn't even stand? With help, I managed two days in bed and felt quite well apart from a raw feeling in the chest, and a suspicion I wasn't breathing properly. This unfamiliar feeling was disturbing; but a couple of weeks later these symptoms disappeared. Nonetheless, my lungs were never the same again.

Prior to this illness, any cold or influenza would disappear in a week, but following this episode I was prone to chest infections which responded only to antibiotics. I was puzzled. Formerly, I had rarely been afflicted with so much as a cough, and now a type of chronic bronchitis had developed — I was continually coughing up foul sputum.

One night I intimated to a doctor that I thought something sinister was occurring. She dismissed my fears and proceeded to ask, 'How do you feel in yourself?' She obviously believed I was seeking attention and saw nothing unusual about my symptoms. Feeling like a raging hypochondriac, I crept out of the surgery. 'Maybe,' I thought, 'everyone in Brisbane suffers with chest problems and they simply ignore the whole thing.'

I should mention here that it pains me to even mildly criticise this doctor. In the 60s, women doctors were rare. Lady Phyllis Cilento was, in my opinion, an absolute genius, and on the occasions I've encountered other women doctors, their empathy and concern have been extremely soothing. Women, in particular, need women doctors.

To return to my story. After two years of frequent chest infections, I awoke about 3am to hear a high pitched whistle coming from my chest. At first I was intrigued, but after two hours the whistling was still sounding, and I realised there would be no more sleep. This nocturnal wheezing continued over the following nights, and the resulting exhaustion (produced by lack of sleep combined with the demands of motherhood) often reduced me to tears.

Following these episodes, I was diagnosed 'Asthmatic' and prescribed both salbutamol and antibiotics. Luckily the antibiotics alone were sufficient because I could never force myself to use the puffer. To my mind, once I used that thing I would be admitting I was an asthmatic. You must remember, during the sixties the general view of asthma was that it was a psychosomatic disease; my pride couldn't handle that. The puffer frightened me — it seemed so abnormal and I have always had an aversion to unnatural things. Perhaps others shared my opinion of the puffer, because most asthmatics at that time tended to use it furtively.

At thirty years of age, I fell pregnant again. From the very first month of that pregnancy I was plagued with chest infections. By the fourth month I'd had three episodes and had completed three courses of antibiotics. A couple of weeks later I succumbed to yet another chest infection. Fears for the baby's health prompted me to forego all antibiotics. Although asthma did not develop, the cough resulting from this infection was unbelievable — it had a definite graveyard quality. My obstetrician said it was probably bronchiectasis but my general practitioner disagreed, stating it was merely bronchitis.

That dreadful cough continued through to the seventh month. My mother said, 'You'll have it till the baby is born for sure. This pregnancy must be taking a lot out of you.' That cough was so embarrassing that I became a virtual recluse.

Then one day everything changed.

A saleswoman for Rawleigh's® products came to my door. She had a range of natural vitamins in stock, and as my eldest son and I were prone to colds, I bought some natural vitamin C — and reeled at the price.

I decided to get my money's worth by asking her some questions about vitamins. She explained that natural vitamins are always more expensive than synthetic. I asked her 'Why is it, that although my son and I take vitamin C tablets regularly, we continually develop chest infections, while my husband who never bothers with vitamins at all, doesn't even catch a cold?'

'Your husband probably eats lots of foods containing vitamin A,' she said. 'Does he like cheese?'

'Does he like cheese? He's practically addicted to it.'

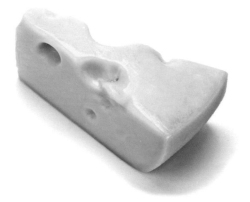

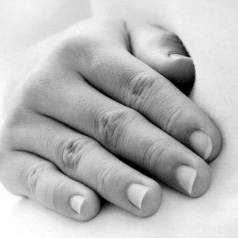

'Well, that could explain it.' She went on to tell me that before commencing with vitamin A herself, she had caught pneumonia twenty-one times and was prescribed antibiotics the size of a ten cent piece. Since she had been using vitamin A she hadn't developed pneumonia once.

Although I was inclined to divide everything she said by three, I was still very impressed by her knowledge of vitamins. Next day I bought some vitamin A from the chemist (much cheaper) and although I took only one capsule per day, the results were amazing. Within three days that cough had disappeared. Continuing with the vitamin until the end of the pregnancy, I suffered no more chest infections, and that horrid graveyard cough never returned.

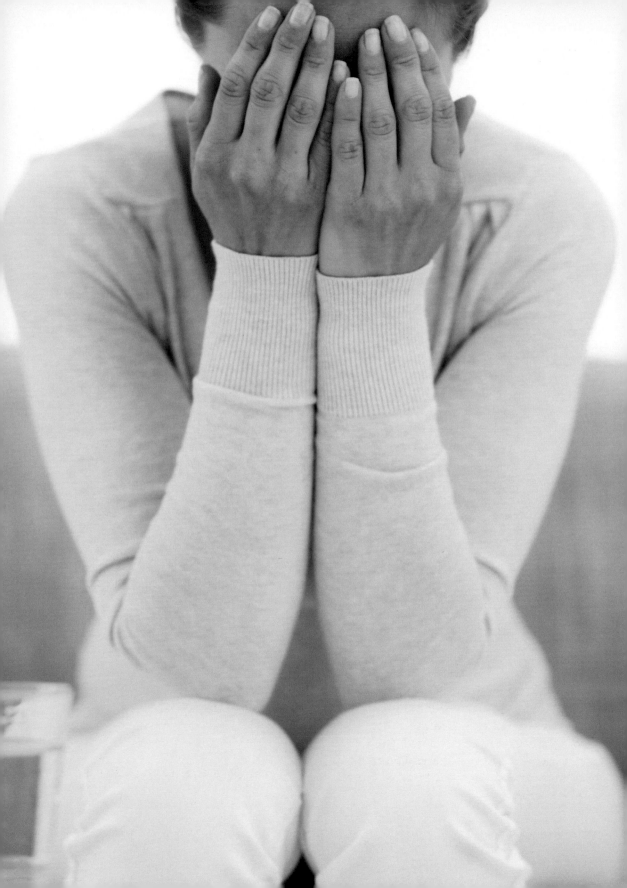

The emotional toll

Bronchitis was now a thing of the past. Whenever I developed a cough, I simply took vitamin A capsules for a couple of days. I found however, as time went on, I was becoming more and more afflicted with asthma. It was particularly troublesome at the change of the seasons when temperatures dropped suddenly.

Although my asthma attacks usually lasted no more than two days, they were stressful, in that they caused chronic tiredness and also emotional problems.

I think most asthmatics try to minimise the emotional trauma. When a person loses control of their life they become depressed. They find themselves unable to function properly. Many fastidious housewives (I wish I was in this category) tell of the anguish of being unable to maintain their homes in what they feel is the necessary state of cleanliness.

For me, it was more a case of feeling inadequate and frustrated whenever I couldn't live up to the expectations of others. From that standpoint, I think asthma could be a definite cause of marital problems. I was doing my best to cope with the children and the housework, when some friends from Rockhampton called in for a visit. It was lovely to see them and I managed to provide refreshments and make conversation, however, by the time they were ready to leave, I was in a haze of exhaustion.

Shortly after their departure, my husband rang. When I told him about the visit, he inquired, 'Did you ask them to stay for tea?' 'No, I didn't think of it.'

'You should have asked them to stay. They came all this way out and you didn't even ask them to stay?'

I was young, immature and terribly upset. I locked myself in the toilet and cried. As those who know me will verify, it takes considerable provocation to induce even a sniffle from me, but on that occasion I felt I'd been pushed over the edge.

I was five months pregnant and although I didn't know it, I was carrying twins. I did suspect that something was different because of the considerable pressure under the rib cage. It felt as if my lungs were being squashed against my ribs. I had also been experiencing asthma symptoms for the previous two or three days, so I was completely miserable.

After crying myself out, I waddled into the kitchen and was absolutely stunned to see my husband standing there. It was only 3pm. 'What on earth are you doing here?' I asked. 'Well, you sounded pretty upset so I thought I'd better come home to check on you.'

I was completely dumbfounded. Jim wouldn't take time off work if Brisbane was hit by an earthquake!

I'm just so lucky to have a loving husband!

I really do feel for asthmatic males. Society expects men to be ever strong, reliable and, in Australia — sporty. Young boys and men who love to compete, and who base their manhood on their sporting prowess, must suffer dreadfully. Australia has many sporting heroes who are asthmatic. What drive and will power they must have to overcome a handicap like asthma.

For 12 months following the birth of the twins, I was extremely healthy (which was just as well because sleep was such a rarity, I was on the verge of collapse). I don't know why I was asthma-free that year. I would never have coped if I had succumbed.

The following year, asthma returned in its previous form. During the winter and change of seasons, I would sleep with the windows in the bedroom closed and if it was cold, have the heater on all night. Keeping the bedroom warm seemed to improve my breathing. The worst hours were from 4.00am until dawn and the resulting lack of sleep often made life difficult.

How Jim tolerated the heat and stuffiness in the bedroom, I'll never know. Thank goodness he can sleep through anything!

One long weekend, the temperatures which had been fairly high up to that point, suddenly plummeted to a low of six degrees. This drop triggered asthma in both myself and our eldest son Danny, then aged 11. At only three years of age, this blonde, blue-eyed boy had been diagnosed with asthmatic bronchitis.

During that freezing holiday break, we two asthma sufferers locked ourselves in a bedroom, turned the heater up, and wheezed away all weekend. At the time we suffered more from 'troublesome' asthma than the 'frightening' variety. I can't even remember using medication apart from Elixophyllin® to help us through the night. We simply felt breathless, miserable, and were confined to bed (Incidentally Elixophyllin® always gave me a giant 'hangover' the next morning).

It wasn't until I was 34 that my first really frightening attack occurred.

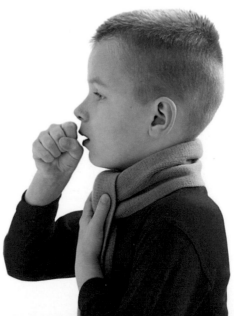

First frightening attack

We had just arrived home from a wonderful holiday at the Gold Coast. I remember sitting in church on Good Friday, wearing my new sundress which revealed a first class tan, and thinking to myself I had never felt fitter or healthier. How quickly things change.

Between 3pm and 9pm, the weather temperature dropped by about 12 degrees. By 9pm I was wondering if I would survive the night. This asthma attack was terrifying. The tightness in my chest was so severe that my lungs felt like blocks of cement and the effort to inhale and exhale was enormous. I should have found the puffer prescribed many years before, but I'd never used it, was still afraid of it, and imagined after all those years it would probably be ineffective.

Being an ex-lifesaver, Jim helped considerably by placing his hands on my rib cage and pumping my lungs as one would a pair of bellows. He couldn't sustain this effort for long. My chest was feeling cold. I gasped, 'Could you fill the hot water bottle for me to cuddle?' Strangely the heat of that bottle seemed to be what was needed, because my breathing improved and I fell asleep. (I am not recommending placing hot water bottles on chests as a suitable treatment for asthma.)

On waking the next morning, I felt so dreadful that I burst into tears. My mother, holidaying with us at the time, appeared shocked to see me so uncharacteristically emotional. In spite of her habitual distrust of doctors, she insisted I visit one immediately.

The doctor prescribed Quibron® tablets; however I received the distinct impression he was not interested in having me as a patient, although he had seemed to welcome our son Danny. I wondered if this difference in enthusiasm had anything to do with our ages. Medical research at the time indicated the future prognosis for children with asthma was very bright, whereas for late-onset asthmatics, it was not good.

Thankfully, for about two years, the Quibron worked well.

After this, a definite pattern seemed to emerge. Attacks were rare in summer or mid-winter. The principal problem times were spring and autumn, and the most potent trigger factor was a sudden drop in temperature. Chest infections also caused asthma, and I was beginning to suspect an allergy to sulphites, because so many attacks occurred on our fish and chips nights. (Sulphites were often sprayed on uncooked potato chips).

For some reason or other, I also developed asthma within two days of returning home from a holiday. Whether this was caused by the time of the year — March to April, or tiredness from the effort of packing and unpacking as well as huge amounts of washing, I don't know.

While the children were at primary school, we spent every holiday period at the Gold Coast. Jim, probably still hankering after his life-saving days, wouldn't consider going anywhere else. I couldn't face camping with small children, so we rented houses or units. Because rental fees double on the Gold Coast during peak seasons, we were forced to go either around February, March or November.

It was a drama writing to all the individual schoolteachers telling them we would be withdrawing the children from their classes for two weeks! Our kids worried about this, but I don't think it did them any harm. Both Jim's and my parents stressed that a family must have a holiday away every year in order to maintain physical and mental health. Holidaying in March probably meant we returned in time for the asthma season and that was why I always succumbed at that time.

When the Quibron ceased working, I visited our new doctor, who seemed very understanding. He prescribed Nuelin® tablets and they were very effective.

The side effects, however, were unpleasant; they made me feel shaky, and if taken after midnight caused headaches the following morning.

I joined a group of young mothers playing weekly squash. I really enjoyed this game because it afforded us a chance to get together and indulge in adult conversation. As the squash courts had glass fronts and a play area for the toddlers, we could manage to have a happy sociable time while still keeping an eye on the children.

It became apparent, though, that unless I took a Nuelin® tablet the night before, I simply couldn't play the game; I had no energy. It appears that as I was getting older, my underlying condition was deteriorating.

Supermarkets were also a problem. How I hated those wide endless aisles with freezing air-conditioning. I did my best to avoid them and always sought out small, non-air-conditioned shops. When my favourite supermarket closed down, I was forced to frequent one of these chilly monsters. The only way I could cope with the weekly grocery order, was to leave the house about 11.30am, buy half the groceries, come home away from the air-conditioning for lunch, then head out again for the remainder of the shopping. I simply couldn't manage the distance around all the aisles — the further I pushed the trolley, the more difficult it was to breathe.

Most people would ask, 'Why didn't you take some medication before leaving home?' The fact is I didn't even think of it. Perhaps my upbringing had something to do with this. My mother abhorred medication, and as children we practically had to write applications in triplicate for permission to take an aspirin.

Attending squash every week was evidently more important than shopping for groceries, which I considered didn't warrant medication!

At age 36, I had been asthmatic for over seven years. Feeling guilty, I told few people of my condition. I think the adages of the 60s: 'Asthma is a psychosomatic disease' and 'An asthmatic child is an unloved child' haunted me. I had combined those opinions and arrived at the conclusion I was both neurotic and unloved. Fortunately, because I didn't consider I had chronic asthma, I could dismiss those thoughts most of the time — until a new pattern emerged.

During spring and autumn, a perpetual month-long tightening of the chest prevented me from inhaling a satisfying quantity of air. Oxygen deprivation brought with it perpetual fatigue and depression: none of the old 'it'll-all-be-over-in-two-days' feeling that I experienced with the more severe attacks. Nuelin® helped me sleep at night, but on the whole it didn't have much effect. Once the month was up, the asthma disappeared.

I began to wonder, when the twins started school, whether I would be able to participate in activities such as tuck-shop. I felt my ill health would make me too unreliable to make a commitment. On days when my asthma was more severe, I would thank God for television, sit the children in front of it and give myself a day in bed. The children enjoyed these days — when I was well, too much viewing was forbidden.

I virtually hibernated from the beginning of winter. At four every afternoon, in order to maintain a warm house, I closed every door and window. I rarely went out on cold nights and constantly had the heater on in the bedroom. Because the dreaded house-dust mite theory had replaced the psychosomatic label as a cause of asthma, I once drove myself into a cleaning frenzy, believing if I eradicated every speck of dust, I would be miraculously cured. It didn't work.

Various other triggers of asthma were soon being espoused — stress, pollen, changes in temperature, exercise, infection, reaction to cats and dogs etc. These 'causes' sounded feasible, except for the fact they all existed in the '40s and '50s when the asthma rate was low. Obviously the triggers were just that; triggers. They could not have been the cause of asthma. Confused, I was even beginning to dread the blooming of the beautiful flowering trees in our area.

Nothing remains the same, however, and future events were to bring about a dramatic alteration in my health and lifestyle. Strangely it was a near disaster which brought about this change.

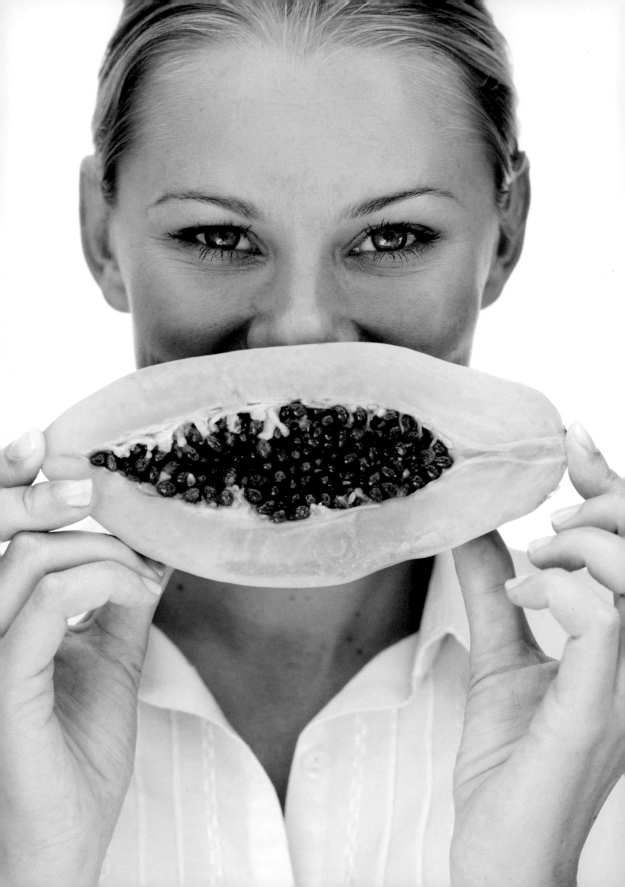

Breakthrough

In my thirty-eighth year, I was hospitalised with a 'virus'. My appendix ruptured — and an exploratory operation led to an emergency appendectomy. Further complications: peritonitis, a blocked bowel, and gangrene kept me in hospital for another two weeks after the surgery. I remember waking at some ungodly hour every morning and thinking, 'How am I ever going to make it through the day?' But for the skill and dedication of an eminent Queensland surgeon, I would not be here. (Incidentally this tall impressive man was very slow to send his bill, and considering the extent of his involvement, his fee was minuscule.)

However, I digress, but I want to demonstrate how this traumatic episode actually produced some good because if I hadn't experienced that illness, I would not have found a cure for my asthma.

About eight weeks after this operation, I was feeling down because I had once again developed 'month-long asthma'. My disappointment was acute as it took a full six weeks to recover, and here I was, mown down again. It all seemed very unfair but looking back, I should have been grateful just to be alive.

Lying in bed one night, wheezing away and feeling sorry for myself, I suddenly pictured asthmatics all over the world, experiencing these same symptoms. I felt a strong empathy with them and vowed to do everything in my power to discover the cause of this illness. It occurred to me that someone developing asthma in adulthood would be much more likely to believe a cure was possible than a person suffering asthma from childhood. Surely long-term asthmatics would be prone to accept their disease as part of life. I made a deal with God. 'You find me a cure for my asthma and I promise I'll publicise it in the hope it will help others.'

Now this is when amazing events occurred. Only two days following this 'deal', Jim arrived home and related a conversation he had with a young co-worker, named Joy. 'How's Marian?' she asked.

'She's improved a lot since the operation,' said Jim, 'but now she's down with asthma.'

Joy replied, 'Asthma is a vitamin A deficiency. Marian needs more vitamin A, but it must be taken with vitamin E. I've heard paw-paw is supposed to be one of the best sources of vitamin A.'

When Jim relayed Joy's message, I believed it immediately. I knew she was very interested in nutrition, and I'd experienced first-hand the benefits of vitamin A for bronchitis. Asthma did seem like a deficiency disease. It did appear to be systemic in that asthmatics often suffer other symptoms besides asthma such as bronchitis, hay fever, rhinitis and eczema. I also remembered Jim telling me of a concept he called the 'trace element theory'. He said a farmer had shown him a field of wheat that was lovely and green except for one small patch, which was yellow. The farmer told Jim the yellow wheat was growing in soil deficient in iron. A small sprinkle of iron in that section would make the whole field green.

It occurred to me that vitamin A could be the missing 'trace element' in asthma — similar to vitamin C in scurvy and iron in the wheat-field.

The following day I went out and bought some vitamin A and synthetic E; (natural E wasn't available in those days). I hadn't a clue what quantity to take, but considered if I had a deficiency, one capsule would probably not be enough, so I took two (total 10,000 units) and one vitamin E (100mg). I also increased my consumption of foods containing vitamin A and carotene, e.g. lamb's fry (not much I must admit), cheese, eggs, carrots, paw-paw, pumpkin, broccoli etcetera.

Within two days I felt marvellous; not a sign of the chronic asthma which had dogged me for the past fortnight. I was really excited and contemplated ringing Joy immediately to thank her for her advice. However, as the whole thing seemed incredible and September (usually a bad month for me) was looming, I decided to wait three months before contacting her.

Bliss! Three months later, and still no asthma.

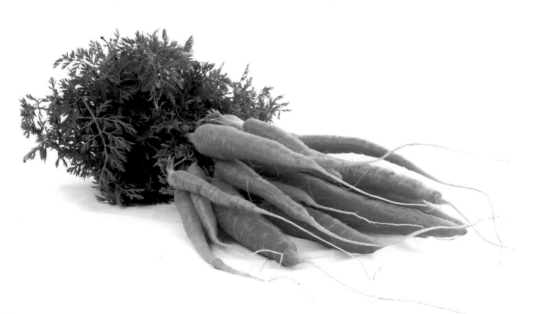

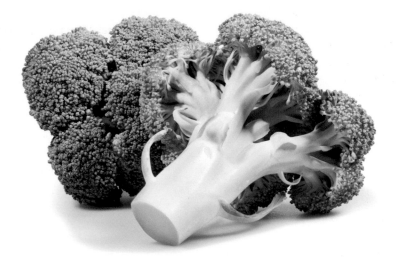

I wasn't taking the vitamins every day, but at the first sign of symptoms, took them immediately and continued for a few days. I tried to tell Joy of this wonderful improvement, only to discover she had left Jim's branch and her whereabouts were unknown. Luckily she rang Jim one day and he told her how thrilled I was with her cure.

Her reply surprised him. 'I didn't say asthma was a vitamin A deficiency,' she said. 'I said, most respiratory problems were a vitamin A deficiency. Asthma is supposed to be an allergy.'

I was shocked to hear Joy had not said asthma was a vitamin A deficiency. Jim however, stuck to his original version, maintaining he'd passed the message on correctly. Well, I thought, what if someone did get their lines crossed and it was all a big mistake; it was a mistake in my favour and I wasn't about to abandon this new found treatment. I hadn't felt so well in years and was sleeping blissfully through the night with windows wide open. I was also back playing squash (requiring no medication), positively roaring around the supermarket and had completely dismissed all thoughts of the stupid house-dust mite. Evening barbeques were no longer avoided and nights out in town (instead of being fearful) were exciting once more.

I was liberated for the first time in ten years.

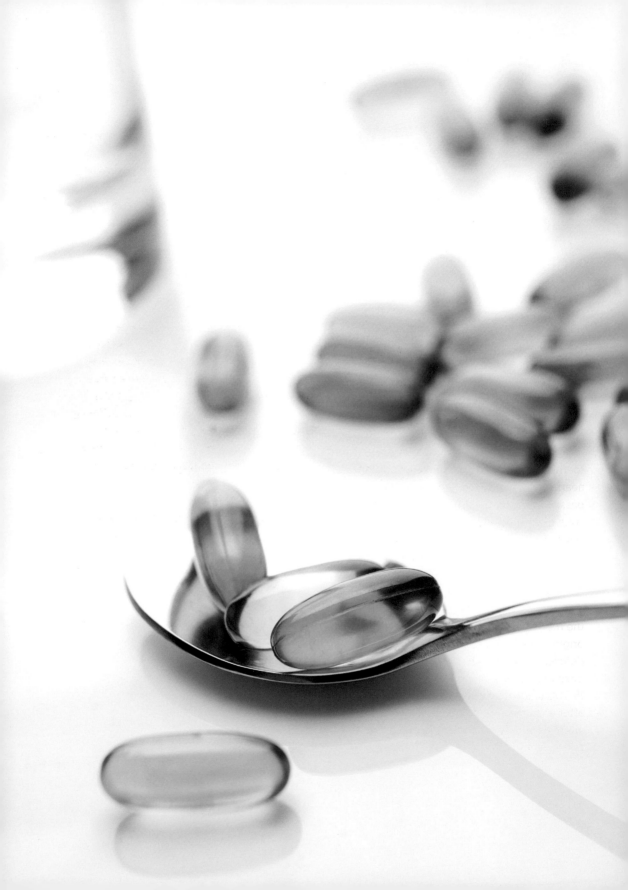

A testing time

This new vitamin treatment was severely tested during the following particularly stressful year. My mother, who had sold her home, wanted to stay permanently with us. As our children ranged in ages from six to fifteen, I felt that adding an eighty-two-year-old to the home would make the situation too difficult.

This problem may not have pressured some people, but being an only daughter (who had never said 'No' to her mother) I found the stress to be intense. I believed I might crack under the strain of so many age groups under the one roof. Thankfully, Jim came to the rescue and organised a lovely unit nearby where she lived happily until she passed away. My point here, though, is that in spite of several months of pressure, I had no symptoms of asthma. It seemed evident that the vitamins also counteracted severe stress.

Three years of excellent health followed. If I noticed a mild wheeze developing in the mornings, I would remind myself of the original premise, 'Asthma is a vitamin A deficiency' and simply increase the dose of A. This always worked. I was taking 15,000 units of vitamin A per day (one capsule after each meal) plus 100mg of vitamin E. The vitamins usually took about twenty hours to take effect.

Everything went swimmingly until one April morning when at 3am I was wakened by a severe asthma attack. Stupidly, I'd allowed myself to run out of Nuelin® tablets, which meant hours of struggling for every breath. My rib cage ached from the effort required to exhale. The next morning, feeling ill, debilitated and shaky, I visited our doctor for a repeat prescription of Nuelin®.

This setback was devastating. My confidence in the vitamin A theory was shattered. I had not missed one dose of vitamins during the previous month. It was unbelievable. How could this happen after three asthma-free years? As any asthmatic will verify, to be free of asthma for 36 months, after suffering regularly for eight years, is nothing short of miraculous. Defeated, I asked myself, 'What was so different about that day from any other day?'

Could it have been the prawns we ate for tea? But we'd eaten fish on other occasions with no ill effect. Could it have been the drop in temperature? But temperatures had dropped countless times over the past three years. Could it have been the 'too cold' air-conditioning at the shopping centre? But this hadn't altered either.

I was completely mystified.

Then I remembered that during the previous two weeks, I had been taking cod-liver oil capsules instead of my usual A (or A+D). Cod- liver oil capsules at that time contained 5,000 units of vitamin A but on inspecting this bottle, I found it was simply labeled '275mg Cod Liver Oil'; no mention of the **quantity** of vitamin A and D in each capsule. In view of this ambiguity, I decided to stop taking it and reverted to my usual capsules.

For the next six weeks, I felt fine. Then, considering it a waste not to use up the old cod-liver oil capsules, I recommenced taking them. Ten days later, another severe attack — once more at 3am. This time I was certain the fault lay with the capsules; they must have been weaker than my usual type.

I rang the chemist at the vitamin company and was surprised when told these particular cod-liver oil capsules contained only 578 units of vitamin A — less than one eighth the usual strength.

What a relief! My faith in the vitamins had been severely tested and I came close to failing the test. I had almost considered giving up completely, but I resumed my normal dosage and another four years of asthma-free living followed.

During those years I found it necessary, during winter, to double the dose of vitamin A in order to maintain normal health. At age 42, I was taking 20,000 units of A, 200mg of Eand an occasional 500mg of vitamin C. At age 44, 30,000 units of A were required and about 500mg of E (in winter). During the summer months I reduced these amounts to almost nil.

On this regime, I experienced seven asthma-free years.

By 1987, Danny (aged twenty-one) and I had been using the vitamins for eight years. During that time, neither he nor I experienced chronic asthma or any acute attacks (apart from the episode with the ultra- weak cod-liver-oil dosage). It was amazing how healthy we were.

Danny stayed with the 10,000 units of A and 200mg of E (when he remembered to take it!) We also took vitamin C if we caught colds. The total vitamin dose was divided into two or three with the capsules taken after meals. We experienced no side effects whatsoever.

Often I marvelled at my good fortune. What a blessing to be able to cope with the responsibilities of mothering six children, and still have enough energy for squash and outings with Jim. I would never have coped without vitamins A and E because I'd have felt perpetually tired and tormented.

A surprising by-product of this treatment was the bonus of never again requiring nasal-drops. Previously a nasal-drop 'junkie' — 1980 was the last year it was necessary for me to purchase these drops. Hay fever attacks also were drastically reduced.

Although I succumbed to upper respiratory tract infections (URTI) with as much regularity as anyone else, amazingly these did not develop into asthma. Many people think if they contract a cold or influenza while taking vitamins, it automatically means the vitamins are not working. They then give up. Viral infections are unavoidable and while in the grip of them, in order to avoid asthma, we should be hitting the vitamins hard.

This is definitely not the time to quit.

Investigating vitamin A

In 1984, I decided it was time to keep my end of the bargain made with God, and publicise my cure. The Sunday Mail published my letter to the editor and gave it top billing. The huge number of phone calls that followed completely overwhelmed me. All callers were inquiring about the dosage I used.

This demonstrated how disillusioned many were with the drug approach to asthma. If the reverse occurred and a fellow asthmatic wrote a letter to the editor extolling the virtues of a new asthma drug, I wouldn't bother ringing him or her, as nothing could surpass the vitamin approach.

As a result of this publicity, there were soon ten of us achieving excellent results with vitamins to control our asthma. I don't know how the other callers fared, however, because although they said they would report back on their progress, very few did. This puzzled me, but after hearing some of them recount the reactions from doctors, relatives and friends, I understood why so many were afraid to try the vitamins.

Many were discouraged with the 'Vitamin A is poisonous' theory. I considered this absolutely ridiculous. How could a vitamin be poisonous?

Lady Cilento (*Medical Mother* p.86) writes:

'This cry of "toxic" by the American FDA and our own echo of the same label have caused many consumers to avoid vitamin A and may have caused serious deficiencies among consumers of all ages. The labelling of "toxic" is now silenced by order of the Federal Court in US, and I only hope that the Australian Health Department will follow suit.'

In view of these scare tactics, it is easy to understand why so many asthmatics were frightened. Still, there were ten brave souls continuing the vitamin treatment. Ironically, Joy, the catalyst of my theory, married a young man who was a severe asthmatic. He also improved amazingly.

Curiosity as to why vitamin A worked so well for asthma prompted me to do some research. One day I found a publication entitled *Improving Your Health with Vitamin A* by Ruth Adams and Frank Murray. This book contained many chapters about the use of vitamin A as a cancer preventative.

'Vitamin A for cancer?' I thought. 'Whatever will they come up with next?' Of course, recent medical research has indicated vitamin A could be a preventative for some cancers, particularly of the lungs and breast. However at that time, I was prepared to dismiss these claims. One section, though, did look interesting — the list of various functions that vitamin A performed in the body, such as: Vitamin A is needed for the health of the eyes, for night vision, colour, and side vision, for healthy linings of all body openings and organs, for resistance to infection, for bone development, to maintain the adrenal glands and the synthesis of certain hormones.

Three of these functions of vitamin A are of particular interest to asthmatics, namely:

1. Resistance to infection.
2. Maintenance of linings of the lungs.
3. Maintenance of adrenal glands and synthesis of certain hormones.

Surely the lungs would be more sensitive to irritants and infection if the linings were not maintained well, and as for the adrenal glands, which hormones did they produce I wondered?

No doubt adrenaline would be one. I knew some asthmatics received injections of adrenaline and the drug salbutamol imitated its action. Wouldn't the adrenal glands produce less adrenaline if they were run down through lack of vitamin A?

Investigating the subject, I discovered two of the principal hormones produced by the adrenal glands, were adrenaline and cortisone. I was excited by this information. (Don't forget we didn't study biology during my school days.) I knew cortisone was given to asthmatics so it occurred to me that maybe a shortage of vitamin A could also mean a shortage of cortisone.

I was so excited that I woke Jim up to tell him about it.

'Come on Marian' he said. 'If you can work that out so can the doctors! If they knew vitamin A worked they'd be giving it to their patients.' 'Maybe they don't believe it would work, so they haven't even tried it', I said. 'I've tried it and I know it works.'

I became even more interested in the study of vitamin A after this, and asked our eldest son, Danny, who was studying Science at Queensland University, to bring home some books from the library.

In one publication *Biochemical Basis of Medicine*, by E.D. Wills, it was demonstrated that rats which were fed diets deficient in vitamin A, were found to have lowered levels of natural cortisone in their bodies. (There didn't appear to be any studies on humans.) If rats are a reliable indicator, how many people are struggling to survive with low levels of cortisone? It appears many of us are deficient in vitamin A.

I found evidence of this in my second, less judgmental, reading of *Improving Your Health with Vitamin A*. It described an examination of 500 autopsy specimens, from five different cities in Canada, which revealed that over 30 per cent of the cadavers had less vitamin A in their livers than when they were born. Eight specimens from Ottawa and 20 per cent from Montreal, showed no vitamin A stores at all.

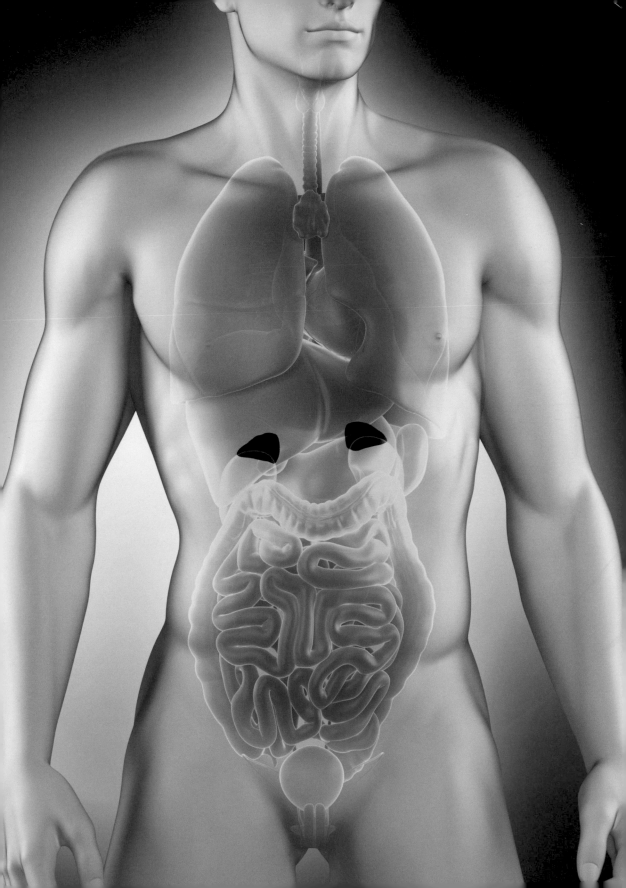

The ages ranged from stillborn to ninety-two, with the majority being over fifty.

Dr T. Keith Murray, when reporting these facts to a nutrition congress held in August 1968, at Puerto Rico, said, 'It is hard to blame diet alone. Even allowing for wastage, cooking losses etcetera it does not seem likely that so many of our population do not get enough vitamin A to maintain their reserves.'

Canadian experts believed there must be something in our environment which is causing us to use up more vitamin A than we can consume, or else our liver stores of vitamin A are being attacked by some substance.

These people suspected pesticides. Did they suspect pesticides because both pesticides and vitamin A are fat soluble, and both accumulate in the liver? (Australians would have higher pesticide levels than Americans because they still use chemicals that were banned years ago in America.)

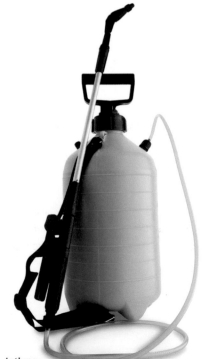

If pesticides or some other chemicals are killing off our vitamin A supplies, or causing us to use up more than we can consume, or preventing absorption of this vitamin, then this could explain why supplementing our diet with extra vitamin A has such a dramatic effect.

To summarise my theory:

• Adrenal glands need vitamin A to keep them healthy and help produce cortisone.
• Cortisone is needed in the lungs to reduce inflammation (one of the chief problems in asthma).
• Pesticides or some other substances are affecting our vitamin A stores.
• If we are suffering from asthma we undoubtedly have insufficient vitamin A to produce enough cortisone, and to maintain the linings of our lungs.

With regard to pesticides — when we consider that humans are at the top of the food chain, the amount of pesticides and heavy metals that we collect in our bodies, is magnified many times. Most pesticides and heavy metals require lengthy periods to fully break down, so each animal or plant that we consume will probably still contain these poisons in its system. As we consume large quantities of all these living products, we naturally absorb large amounts of poisons.

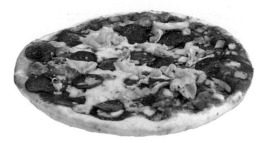

The quantity of food additives present in today's processed foods, and absent from our ancestors' diets, should also be considered as possible destroyers of vitamin A. Are we sure these chemicals are completely safe? Are we certain they are not destroying vitamins or causing us to require more?

Authors, Ross Meillon and Chris Reading claim that many vitamin deficiencies are caused by allergies to food. They claim food allergies prevent the absorption of vitamins. (*Relatively Speaking* p.100). Could this factor also be affecting asthmatics?

Other contributors to *The Complete Book of Vitamins* have more to say on the subject. The U.S. Army Research Institute of Environmental Medicine, testing on rats, proved that when the temperature drops, the body uses less of the available vitamin A and stores more away.

I can't understand why nature dictates the liver should grab so much vitamin A right when we need it. Maybe it's stockpiled for an anticipated attack of winter influenza?

These researchers also stated:

'As the weather gets colder, the consumption of vitamin A should increase to help maintain the same level of health during the winter as in the warmer months.'

When we consider this information on pesticides and food additives and accept that they all increased enormously after World War II, it does seem that a connection can reasonably be made between these factors and the incredible increase in asthma since that time.

Whatever the cause of this vitamin deficiency my belief is this Asthma is a vitamin A deficiency. Vitamin A must always be taken with vitamin E (to protect the A) and some vitamin C is usually required as well.

Of course, the most common response from those hearing this theory for the first time is,

'You shouldn't go around saying things like that. Just because vitamin A works for you, doesn't mean it will work for everyone.'

My answer to this is 'It doesn't only work for me; it works for many others as well and why shouldn't it work for everyone?' Where has it ever been demonstrated that vitamin C will cure scurvy in some, but not in others? Whoever heard vitamin B12 only occasionally controls pernicious anemia? The same could be said for the other diseases controlled by vitamins:

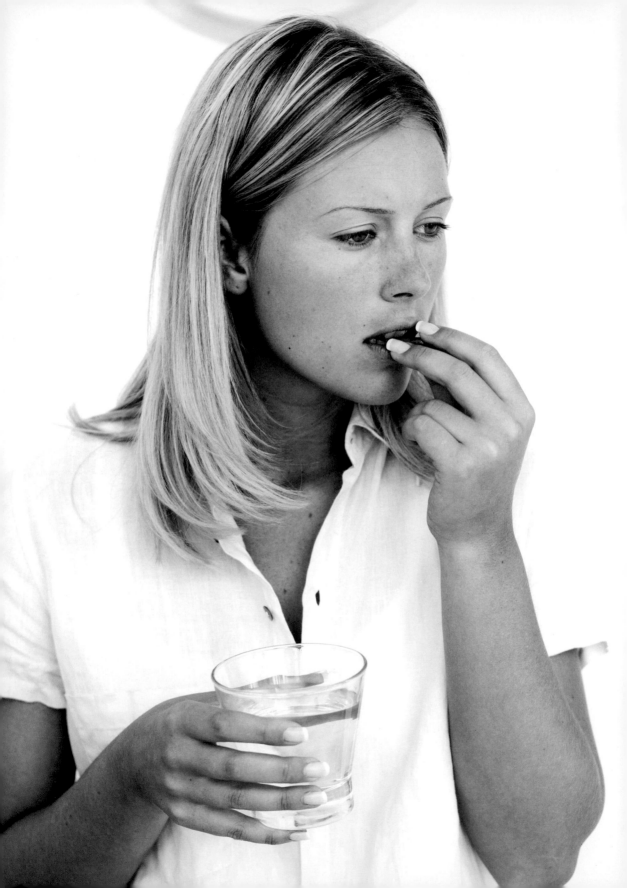

Admittedly, most of these illnesses are seldom seen in Australia, but pernicious anemia is common (I personally know of six cases). The point is we do not have to live in a third world country or belong to a low socio-economic group to suffer a nutritional disease.

Regarding asthma, though, I believe the only reason vitamin A might not work for 'everyone' is simply that 'everyone' hasn't tried it. As previously stated, I've seldom known this treatment to fail, if adhered to correctly.

I once spoke of this vitamin treatment to a woman involved in fundraising for childhood diseases. Her reaction surprised me.
'I don't want you to take this the wrong way, dear, but I don't think anyone is going to believe in that theory of yours.'

'Why not?'

'Well,' she said, 'it's just too simple.'

She seemed a very kind person so I didn't labour the point, but as a good friend of mine said, 'Some of the world's greatest discoveries have been very simple.'

Because asthma has become such a complicated disease, some people find it impossible to believe a simple approach would have any effect. I believe it's a mistake to think like that. Scurvy was once considered one of the biggest killers of all time, and look how that was dealt with.

As far as asthma is concerned, we should also remember there are drug companies with vested interests. Would they want to know of a simple treatment for this disease?

It is important for those who have found relief with this 'too simple approach' to hold fast to our belief, and refuse to back down under the pressure.

Eventually we will win.

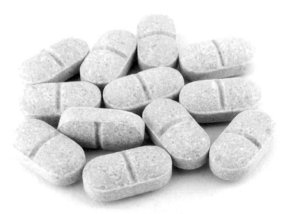

Negative reactions from doctors and drugs

Along with other sufferers and parents, I attended an asthma seminar in 1986. The information shared at that gathering was both disturbing and enlightening.

In one instance, a mother's anger overflowed when the lecturer told of a death in a hospital ward.

'A nine-year-old boy died,' said the doctor, 'because of the stress caused by his estranged parents arguing over who was to take him home for the holiday break.'

'Are you blaming the parents for his death?' the woman snapped, 'How come he died in hospital with every treatment available?' The lecturer quickly changed the subject.

A dark-haired young man, sitting near the front, leapt to his feet and demanded that future doctors be trained to 'please please listen to mothers'.

Another woman told how her child had been on Intal® to prevent asthma and she had suffered as many attacks on the drug, as off it. When asked, 'What does asthma mean to you?' an attractive, but obviously tired, middle-aged woman said: 'Asthma means poverty to me. We have six asthmatics in our family.'

Here was the tall, burly doctor standing in front of a table laden with pharmaceutical products. Never have I seen so many medications and accessories for one disease! Could some of the anger in that room be attributed to fear of commercial exploitation?

Similar feelings surface when we observe the reactions of medical practitioners to any natural approach to asthma. The simpler treatment is either dismissed with a laugh or a warning is issued on the dire consequences of following anything but the orthodox line.

The mother of a 16-year-old asthmatic said, 'When I asked the doctor if there was anything more natural my daughter could try, he replied, "Do you want her to die?"' Later this same mother watched another doctor administer so much salbutamol to her daughter, that the girl lost consciousness.

Another asthma sufferer, after informing his doctor he intended to take vitamins, was told, 'Vitamins don't work! That medical matriarch (referring to Lady Cilento and her book Medical Mother) who pushes them all the time, is a quack. The only reason she's lived so long is longevity runs in her family.'

The strangest comment I heard attributed to a health professional was 'Vitamins can damage your lungs.' This was told to the mother of a four-year-old asthmatic who attended a kindergarten in Ipswich where 13 of the 25 children suffered asthma.

Everyone knows drugs are sometimes essential, but surely simple, natural and safer methods should always be tried first, especially where small children are concerned.

Any housewife will agree that to remove a stain from a garment, you begin with gentle treatments to avoid damaging the fabric; severe methods are only tried when everything else has failed. Why is this not done with asthma? Why do we find four-year-olds on cortisone?

A former pharmaceutical salesman told me he often asked doctors, 'Would you give steroids to your four-year-old?'

The orthodox treatment for asthma demands too much of the patient and too much of the general practitioner. Some asthmatics are taking up to forty puffs of one medication or another every day. How do they cope?

The problem is, should anything go wrong, it is too easy to blame the patient for not remembering to take all his or her medicine; the parent for neglecting to give it to the child or even the doctor for not stressing the importance of each medication.

Surely there could be nothing more painful than to be blamed for the death or severe illness of a loved one. It would be similar to blaming parents when a child drowns in a swimming pool. Haven't these people suffered enough?

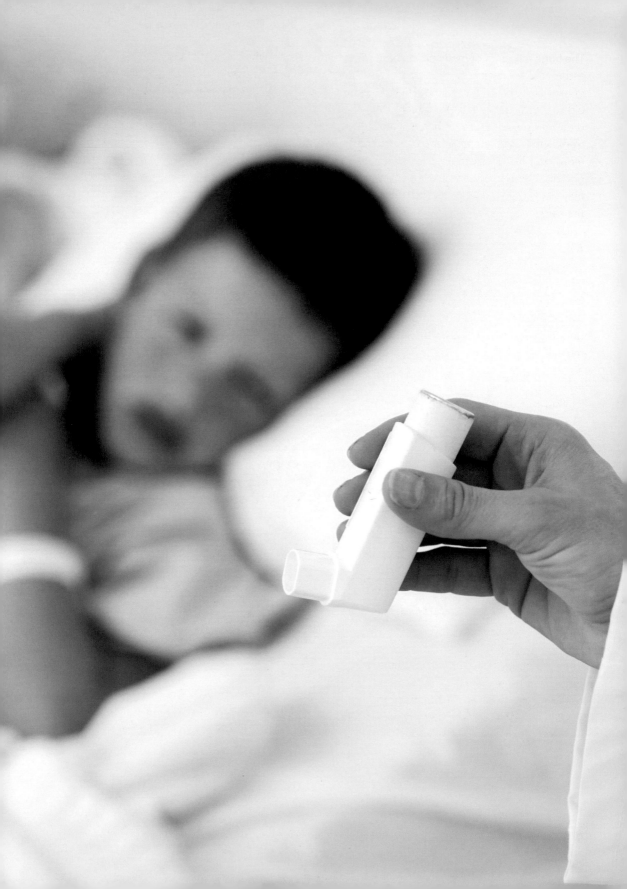

The huge amounts of medication some asthmatics are taking must interfere with their quality of life. A mother told me her 13-year-old son was unable to sit for a technical drawing exam because his hands were still trembling from the nebuliser he'd used that morning. I also received an email from a grandmother who was worried her grandson may have to abandon his dentistry studies for the same reason.

A good friend, Beverley, described another case. Her lively little four- year-old niece, who was very proud of her ability to tie bows, offered to demonstrate this art for her aunt. However, she was unable to tie the ribbon because her hands were shaking too much. Like the 13-year- old boy, this tot had also been attached to a nebuliser. Beverley said, 'It was very sad to hear the child say, "Sometimes I can't do it, Aunty."'

(Imagine the outcry if vitamin A caused side effects like that!)

Lately the trend seems to be more towards inhaled cortisone as a preventative, and away from bronchodilators. While the dangers of over-exposure to bronchodilators are receiving more attention, the belief in the safety of inhaled cortisone is dubious and will probably be resisted by concerned users who have heard of the detrimental effects of long-term cortisone use.

The medical profession is not infallible. When I was growing up in Central Queensland, I asked my mother why the nurses from the local hospital were practically the only women in town who smoked cigarettes. My mother replied the doctors encouraged the nurses to smoke because it was good for their nerves.

I found that difficult to believe. Surely no doctor would encourage smoking? It was common knowledge cigarettes were addictive and I'm sure the term 'smoker's cough' was well known. Admittedly, at that time, no one knew anything of the fatal outcomes.

When a person deals constantly with sickness, does he or she lose interest in maintaining natural good health? The man who discovered vitamin C, Dr Albert Szent-Györgyi seemed to feel this could be a problem:

'Present medicine is lop-sided. As a medical student I had to listen no end to lectures on disease, but cannot remember one on health, full health!' (*Vitamin C Against Cancer*, Dr Szent-Györgyi, who won a Nobel Prize in 1937.)

As to the inhaled cortisone question, I don't pretend to understand the medical aspect. All I know is when I asked my doctor many years ago for a repeat of cortisone cream for my hands, he asked me how long I'd been using it. I said 'Oh, on and off for 13 years.'

He replied, 'You can't keep using that forever, you know.'

What puzzles me is this. If it's not safe to continue using cortisone on my hands, why would it be safe to keep pumping it into my lungs?

Unexpected asthma attack

When Danny was 21 he suffered an unexpected asthma attack. It was his first relapse since commencing the vitamins at age 14. Thankfully he recovered completely in three days, but I soon succumbed to probably the same virus. I didn't suffer the constant asthma that afflicted Danny; mine was breathing difficulties during the night.

The first thing I did was to increase the vitamin A, but to no avail. I doubled the dose; still no improvement. Increasing the vitamin E had no effect. Next I tried changing brands — still no difference. Something was wrong.

Devastated, I was convinced the vitamins had let me down. I was forced to take Theodur® nightly and, although it was more effective than the Nuelin®, it still caused side effects, e.g. shakiness in the legs, hyperactivity and slight nausea. Although these effects lessened as the days passed, I was worried.

In a newspaper article, Lady Phyllis Cilento claimed the only effective treatment against viral infection, was vitamin C. As I was convinced I had a virus, I followed the good doctor's advice, and added one teaspoon of vitamin C powder (Calcium Ascorbate) to my usual vitamins. I took the vitamin C as one would a course of antibiotics,

e.g. one teaspoon three times a day for five days. (In retrospect, it seems a high dose of vitamin C but as diarrhea didn't develop, I mustn't have overdone it.)

Within 24 hours I no longer required the Theodur® and was saved from resorting to stronger medication. To this day I still take a half a teaspoon of vitamin C powder per day.

I wrote to the asthmatics who had maintained contact (who were taking the vitamins) and explained why I had added vitamin C to my regime.

Around this time Queensland, Australia, was dubbed the 'Asthma Capital of the World.' The incidence of the disease in children was 50 per cent higher in Queensland than in Tasmania. The Asthma Foundation reported the death rate from asthma had more than doubled. In 1975 approx. two per 100,000 people died, in 1985 it had reached five per 100,000.

The Emeritus Consultant Physician at the Royal Adelaide Hospital, Dr Munro-Ford said 'These are grim figures indeed when one considers the multitude of new drugs now available, the increased awareness and patient understanding about their disease and the existence of active, well-endowed asthma foundations in every State.'

There was a time when asthma was not considered fatal. What has changed?

If you are over 65, can you recall any asthma sufferers at your school?

When my children were at school in Brisbane, there were 5 or 6 in each class who were asthmatic.

At 45 years of age, I was besieged with problems again, caused chiefly I believe, by that incurable disease — AGE.

When we reach forty-five, our bodies undergo changes. One of these is the necessity to wear reading glasses. Almost every woman I knew had to rummage in her handbag for her glasses to read a restaurant menu. On a few hilarious occasions, only one in our group remembered her spectacles and when the menu arrived, that one pair had to be passed around the entire table.

Maybe there was a connection between all those women needing spectacles and the body's ability to absorb vitamin A?

I should have realised the quantity of vitamins sufficient for a 38-year-old, would not meet those of a 45-year-old. As the body ages, it tends to lose some of its ability to absorb nutrients, and as the gift of sight is very closely associated with vitamin A, I wondered about this.

Why didn't I consider it when asthma struck once more?

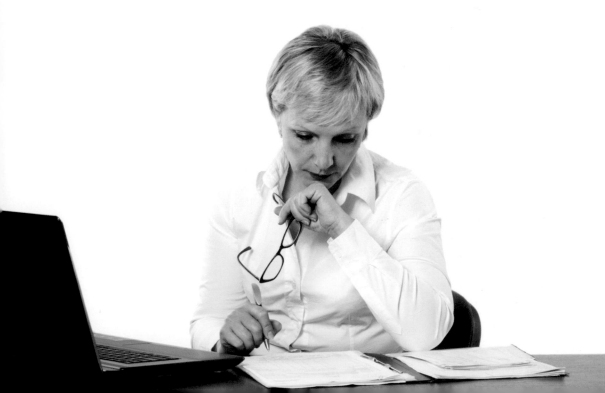

This time, it wasn't only disturbed nights; this was the real thing.

During a family outing at Sanctuary Cove (a resort near the Gold Coast) I experienced the disabling effects of asthma. It was a beautiful autumn day, crisp and sunny, the sea and sky shimmering. One could not imagine ill health when surrounded by such clear air.

We decided to wander along the boardwalk overlooking the yacht harbour. That's when it hit me. Even to walk the short distance, from one side of the boardwalk to the other, was beyond me!

Because the asthma of the previous year appeared to be viral related, I assumed the same of this new outbreak. Therefore, I increased the vitamin C to three teaspoons per day — no improvement whatsoever; doubling the vitamin A to 40,000 units and increasing the E to 500mg produced no results either. This time I believed I was truly beaten.

Another day during this distressing period remains in my memory, primarily because it illustrates the anguish suffered by very severe asthmatics.

We had promised the twins some guinea pigs for their birthday; (must have had rocks in our heads!). We sallied forth to the pet shop, which had a long cement ramp from the footpath to the door.

Normally I'd have bounded up such a ramp, but on this day, the struggle to negotiate that incline was enormous. I suddenly believed I could see the future. I knew, should this condition remain, I would be lucky to last another decade. 'How long could a heart sustain this effort?' I wondered. Deep sadness prompted the additional thought, 'Life would scarcely be worth living anyway.'

For ten days, (while taking Theodur® at night) I experimented with the vitamins, attempting to find the correct ratio. The future looked bleak as I could see no alternative to either constant use of a puffer, cortisone, or probably both.

Before ringing the doctor, I decided to make one last attempt with the vitamins. In her book *Medical Mother*, Lady Cilento set out a vitamin regime for the treatment of chronic respiratory tract infections. She mentioned that asthma would benefit from this regime.

In the past I regarded her recommendation of 60,000 units of vitamin A as completely 'over the top'. However, I was desperate. Surely no harm would befall a person taking larger amounts for only a few days?

In the good Australian tradition, I 'gave it a go' and took six 10,000 unit capsules per day. Within two days of commencing this larger dose, I felt marvelous. Even though I stayed on the high dosage for three months, I suffered no side effects. By the beginning of June I was in fine spirits, and the remainder of the year included some freezing, but magical days and nights at Expo 88.

I couldn't help thinking of Mrs Leone Edwards, who died of an asthma attack shortly before the opening of Expo. Ironically, her husband Sir Llew Edwards, was the driving force behind this international exhibition where millions enjoyed themselves.

I wrote to the other asthma sufferers, and told them of my new dosage, and included the following table:

At Age 45

Temperature	Vitamin Dose
4° to 8° (min)	60,000 i.u. A, 500mg E, 3 teaspoon C
8° to 15°	30,000 i.u. A, 500mg E, 1 teaspoon C
15° and over	20,000 i.u. A, 500mg E, half teaspoon C
Very hot days	Omit altogether unless you react to high humidity

Lady Cilento wrote:

'Large doses, 60,000 to 90,000 units, are sometimes needed for chronic respiratory infections. These doses are non-toxic when taken with Vitamin E and C and not continued for more than three months; then reduce dose to 40,000, but do not cease.'

Not being a chronic respiratory infection sufferer, I sometimes omit vitamins during hot weather. This seems to me a good idea, just in case I did accumulate too much during winter. When the weather turned cool, I re-commenced the higher doses and this enabled me to play squash throughout the year with not so much as a wheeze.

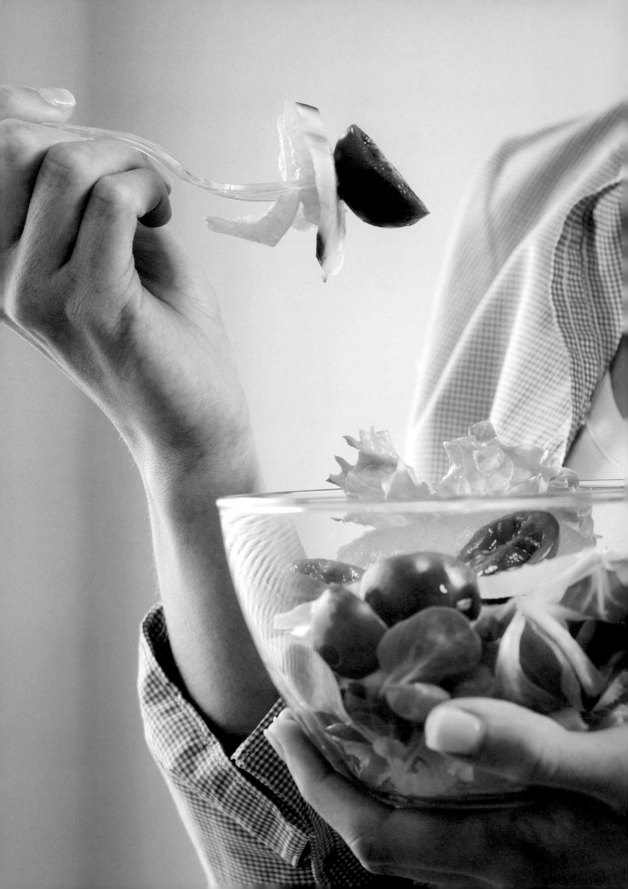

The king of vitamins

It is not easy to obtain a sufficient daily intake of vitamin A from our usual diet.

Vitamin A Foods

Listed below is a chart containing various foods and their accompanying vitamin A levels: (from *Clinical Dietetics and Nutrition*)

You will note: 'Only one third of beta-carotene is absorbed and only one half of what is absorbed is converted to vitamin A. Thus only one sixth of dietary beta- carotene is converted to vitamin A.'

Vitamin A or carotene content of various foods

Food	Vitamin A i.u. per 100gram	Food	Carotene(*) i.u. per 100gram
Halibut-liver oil	4,000,000	Carrots-mature	20,000
Cod-liver oil	200,000	Spinach	13,000
Liver, sheep	45,000	Beet leaves	11,000
Liver, ox	15,000	Carrots,young	10,000
Liver, pig	5,000	Cress	8,000
Liver, calf	4,000	Kale	8,000
Butter	3,500	Sweet potato	6,000
Cheese		Watercress	5,000
(whole fat)	1,500	Apricot	2,000
Eggs, hen	1,100	Lettuce	2,000
Kidney, ox	1,000	Tomato	1,200
Salmon, canned	250	Peach	800
Milk, summer	150	Brussels sprouts	700
Herrings, fresh	100	Cabbage	500
Milk, winter	75	Maize, yellow	350
Beef or mutton	20		

(*) Divide by 6

The second column in the above chart mentions the top carotene containing foods and gives the amount of units contained in 100 grams. As carotene has to be converted into vitamin A within the body, the actual amount extracted from the carotene would be much lower than indicated.

Therefore in order to ascertain the quantity of vitamin A received from each fruit and vegetable, **we are required to divide the figures in the right hand column, by six.**

Carotene is converted into vitamin A primarily in the **intestinal wall**.

PLEASE NOTE: Diabetics are incapable of converting carotene into vitamin A. (*Clinical Dietetics and Nutrition*).

As we can see, unless we take cod or halibut-liver oil or eat some type of liver at least once a week, our diet would probably not supply the 1988 Recommended Daily Allowance of 5,000 units of vitamin A.

Why then are we continually being told vitamin supplements are not necessary?

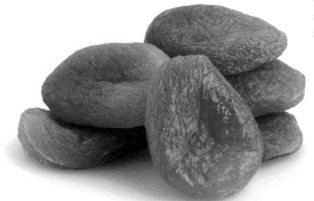

Michael B. Sporn, M.D. of the American National Cancer Institute, believes we should be concerned about consuming too little vitamin A. He claims there is a definite connection between cancer rates and low levels of vitamin A. I quote his statement from *The Complete Book of Vitamins*:

'The data at hand clearly indicates that any human population at risk of cancer, should not be allowed to remain in a vitamin A deficient state.'

Are we at risk of cancer?

Do you recall Dr Linus Pauling, the double Nobel Prize winner? He argued **against** a move in America to restrict vitamin A capsules to 10,000 units.

A further quote from the publication *Improving your Health with Vitamin A*, p. 69, indicates how the body uses natural vitamin A: 'Whatever you don't need on a daily basis is stored in your liver.'

Children need much less vitamin A than adults. Lady Cilento suggests cod liver oil as a source of vitamin A for children — 1 teaspoon to 1 tablespoon a day according to age. (Surely she meant Hypol®, Scott's Emulsion® or cod-liver oil capsules!) In her book *Medical Mother* p.87, she suggests the Vitamin E dose for children should be 50mg to 100mg.

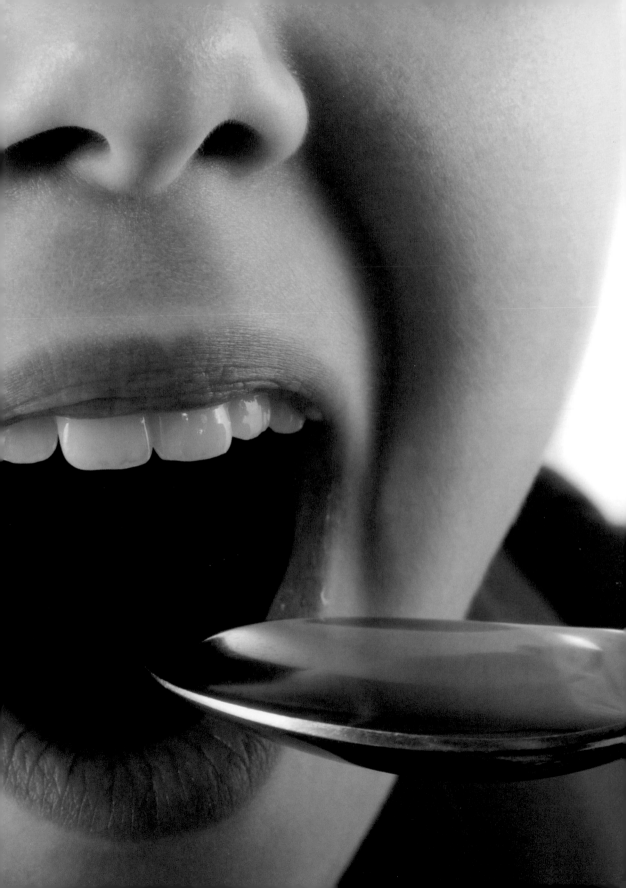

Lady Cilento also included a paragraph on vitamin A overdose in her book *Vitamin and Mineral Deficiencies*:

'Too much vitamin A can be toxic, causing thinning hair, sore lips, bruising, nose bleeds, headaches, blurred vision, flaky itching skin, painful joints and bones. But for toxicity to occur, you would have to take over 100,000 units a day for a long time. These symptoms can be prevented by generous doses of vitamin C — say 1000mg a day — but even if vitamin C and E are not taken, the symptoms completely disappear in a few days after ceasing vitamin A'.

A chart of over-dose symptoms distributed by **Bio-Concepts**, Kelvin Grove, Qld., states that an acute toxic dose would be 250,000 units per day. A chronic overdose would be 60,000 to 90,000 units per day for six months, so they are more conservative than Lady Cilento. To emphasise individual reactions to dosages: a Brisbane nutritionist told me that she suffers symptoms on only 30,000 units, yet I take 60,000 for more than three months with no side-effects.

It bears reiterating; there must be wide variations in each person's daily requirement for this vitamin, and we must also keep in mind any **overdose is reversible within a few days of ceasing the vitamin**.

The American Recommended Daily Allowance for Vitamin A is alarmingly low, particularly when we consider Dr Sporn's assertion on the relationship between cancer rates and vitamin A deficiency.

They recommend 5,000 units for a boy of 11 and a man over 51, regardless of the difference in age, body-weight, exercise levels, stress levels and general state of health.

Remember this: 5,000 does not just represent the level of vitamin A received from supplements, it includes the total amount of vitamin A received in the daily food as well.

At least the American Daily allowance recognises pregnant and lactating women require more vitamin A than others. They add another 1,000 units for pregnancy and an extra 2,000 units for breast- feeding to the female recommendation of 4,000 units. ('Foundations of Normal and Therapeutic Nutrition').

Not only do vitamin needs vary from individual to individual but some people, like my husband, are perfectly healthy without the help of any vitamin supplements whatsoever while I require, during winter, at least 40,000 units **per day**.

In her book *Vitamins and your Health*, nutritionist Ann Gildroy writes, in the time of scurvy, although the sailors were eating identical foods, many succumbed to the disease and died, while others remained unscathed. Food for thought?

The founder of Vitamin Therapy, Dr Abram Hoffer, helps illustrate this point. In 1951, Dr Hoffer gave large amounts of vitamin B3 to hallucinating patients, even though they were not suffering from the vitamin B3 deficiency disease, pellagra. They recovered from their psychosis. He believes they simply had a much larger than usual requirement for this vitamin. (From *Dr Atkins' Nutrition Breakthrough*).

Dr Hoffer's experiment was the forerunner of Orthomolecular Medicine. Dr Linus Pauling coined the term 'orthomolecular' which means the importance of making the biochemical environment just right.

Frankly, I believe we should ignore most of the The American Recommended Daily Requirements and Dr. Irwin Stone, obviously agrees:

'The Food and Nutrition Board has been reducing the RDA for ascorbate (Vit. C) with each new edition of their book 'Recommended Dietary Allowances'. In 1958, the adult RDA for ascorbate was 75mg, in 1968 it went down to 60mg, and in their latest exploit in 1975, it lost another 25% and became 35mg. If the Food and Nutrition Board continues whittling away at its present rate, the RDA (for Vit.C) will be zero by the year 2000'.

(The Complete Book Of Vitamins)

(Dr. Stone was a little pessimistic as the RDA for vitamin C is still around 35mg).
The vitamin A chart recommends liver as a good source of vitamin A. While liver does contain large amounts of A, it also has a tendency to collect high levels of pesticides and other poisons.

I quote from *Toxicology of Pesticides*:

'Partly because of their great importance for bio-transformation and excretion, the liver and kidneys often show high concentrations of foreign chemicals.'

I wonder if it's wise to consume large amounts of liver, if, as also mentioned in this publication, 'DDT is found in virtually everyone in the general population of USA and other countries.'

We can be sure beasts are also affected, although lamb's fry, being from a young animal, should be the safest.

Every one, from the sailor in bygone ages to the asthmatic of today, is different, and we all require varying amounts of nutrients. Some seem to need large amounts of vitamin A to remain healthy, while others do not.

My advice is — listen to your body.

It doesn't know its supposed daily requirements — it only knows what it **needs**.

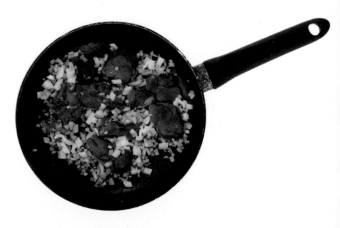

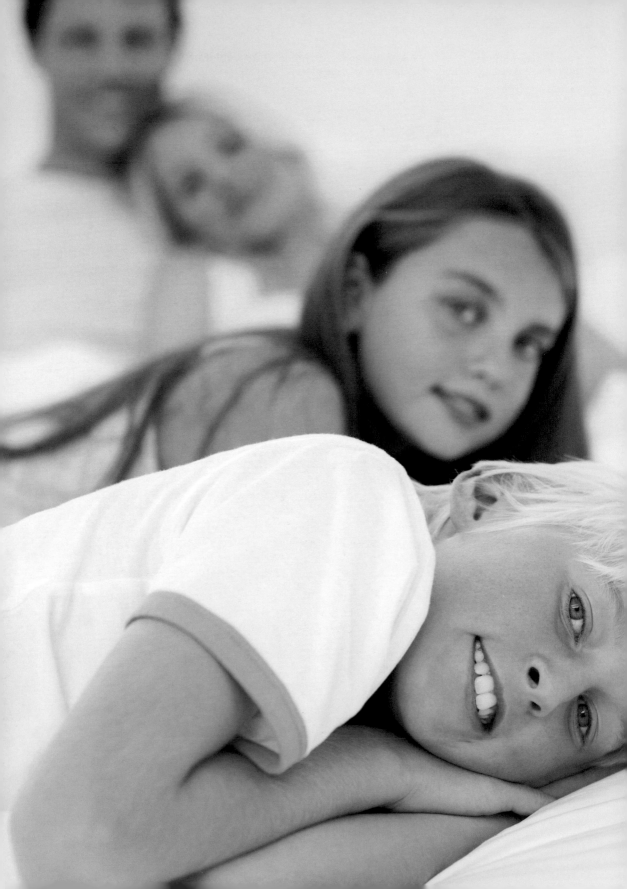

Antibiotics and childhood asthma

Research has indicated a connection between the use of antibiotics and an increased risk of developing asthma. A study carried out by the Henry Ford Hospital in the United States has found that children given an antibiotic (usually penicillin) under the age of six months, more than doubled their likelihood of developing asthma by the age of seven.

The above results were presented at the European Respiratory Society's conference in Vienna in 2003.

Another study carried out in New Zealand and published in the *Journal of Clinical and Experimental Allergy 1999*, researched broad-spectrum antibiotics taken through the first year of life. Those children given multiple courses of antibiotics were four times more likely to develop asthma than a child who had never taken antibiotics. The question here is 'Which comes first, the chicken or the egg?' Were these children genetically prone to asthma or born with very low vitamin A levels so therefore required more antibiotics and would have gone on to develop the illness anyway, or did the antibiotics affect the gastrointestinal tract, harming the development of the immune system, and thereby causing asthma?

One of the New Zealand researchers, Professor Crane from Otago University called for caution, saying the results cannot be taken as definitive. 'On the other hand,' she says, 'the results are plausible. Broad-spectrum antibiotics came into clinical usage in the 1960s, and their increased use coincides with the time trends for the increasing prevalence of asthma. There is a plausible mechanism, namely that broad-spectrum antibiotics may alter and reduce bowel flora and thus switch off the immunological signals that these gut bacteria send to the developing immune system.'

It all sounds very complicated. Dr. Alan Greene MD FAAP suggests on his web site that if it is necessary for children to have antibiotics, parents should ask for the most narrow- spectrum choice that would work and the child should also be given probiotics to replace the beneficial bacteria.

After reading this research, I remembered how, twenty years ago I'd read in a publication in the Biology Library at Queensland University that antibiotics could damage a part of the intestines responsible for the absorption of vitamin A. I thought at the time, this could be a reason asthmatics need extra vitamin A.

As I couldn't remember the title or author of this book, I decided to do a 'Google' search to find more information. You guessed it. There are many articles on the internet about antibiotics reducing absorption of vitamins K, E, B3, B6, B7 and C, but no mention of them affecting vitamin A.

I don't know what to make of this. It seems practically every asthmatic I've known has taken many courses of antibiotics. You would think if antibiotics reduce the absorption of vitamin E, they would also affect vitamin A, as these two vitamins are usually found together. Still I can't find any evidence to support this theory, apart from my memory of reading the article in the Biology Library.

If it is true, and the ability to absorb vitamins A and E is reduced by antibiotics, it could explain why asthmatics need to increase their intake of these vitamins, and it could also explain why so many researchers are making a connection between asthma and antibiotics.

I guess the problem here is some people might take this too far and reject antibiotics when they are urgently required to fight a fatal infection.

Another theory on childhood asthma has come from some respiratory specialists who have attributed the increase to couples having smaller families. They reason modern children are not being exposed to as many germs, so their immune systems are less well developed than those from large families or in child-care.

Like many previous explanations, this sounds feasible. However, if this theory is true, asthma should have been more common in schools of the 1940s and 1950s. Admittedly, most families were larger then, but there were still many small families like Jim's and mine and plenty of first-borns and only children. Yet asthma was practically unknown.

Perhaps today's youngsters from large families or in child-care, appear to have better immune systems because their mothers might try harder to boost these children's immunity. Child-care centres reject sick children while mothers of large families know if one sibling falls ill, you can bet they all will!

As mentioned earlier, I popped vitamin C tablets into anyone with the sniffles and I've heard mothers of other large families and those using child-care, say they do the same thing. Perhaps these extra vitamins improve the immunity of these children.

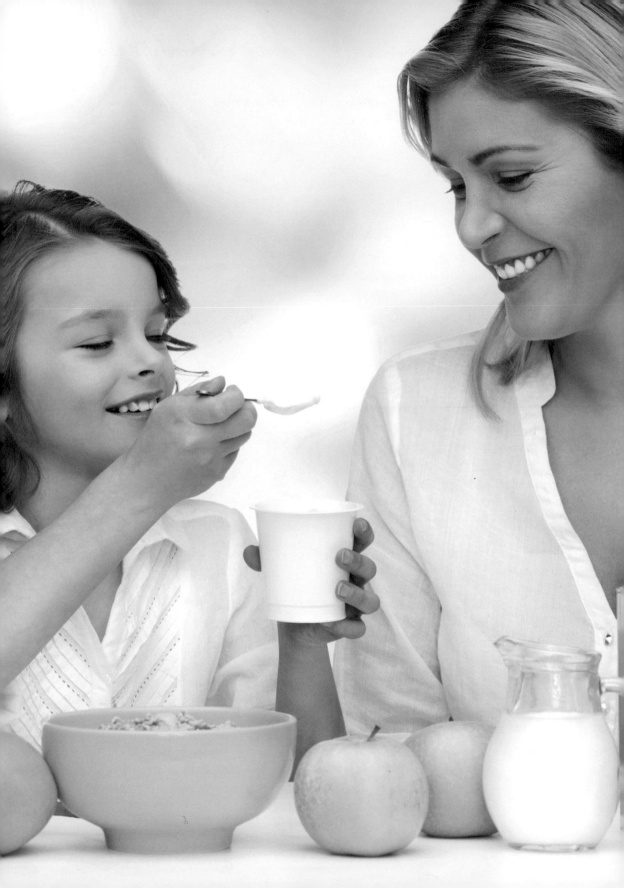

If antibiotics affect the ability to absorb many vitamins, then our modern diet would not be helping to address this issue. Our smaller intake of dairy products must result in lower vitamin A levels. Many of us have substituted margarine for butter; we eat different desserts; and we tend to eat lighter breakfasts.

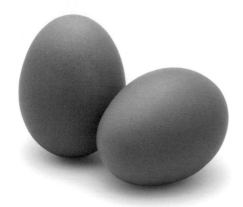

Because earlier refrigeration was so inefficient, children in the '40s and '50s rarely enjoyed treats like ice-cream. Most would have eaten only homemade desserts — for example stewed fruits and baked custards, or fruit topped with boiled custard or cream. The custard would have been made with fresh milk and eggs (probably from the family's own hens) and the cream skimmed from the top of the milk.

One of my mother's prized recipes, 'Queen Pudding', used four eggs. This would equal about 3,200 units of vitamin A, plus other important nutrients. Another favourite, 'Bread and Butter Pudding', included three eggs and real butter on the bread. (Butter is an excellent source of vitamin A). Today, supermarket ice-cream with fruit or chocolate topping is probably the most common dessert.

Most families in the '50s, also had what was called 'lamb's fry night' (which was most unpopular with the children). Liver in the form of beef liver and lamb's fry is very high in vitamin A. Recently nutritionists have been stating that Australian liver is safe to eat. The previous belief that it contained high amounts of toxins has now been found to refer to European and North American liver. 'Australian pastures are clean. Northern hemisphere stock is barn/stall fed on growth hormones and grain fodder. The grains have been sprayed with herbicides and insecticides.' (*From It Could Be Allergy and It Can be Cured*) When we combine the above diet with the whopping spoonfuls of cod liver oil given to most children, it is obvious these earlier generations consumed considerably more vitamins A, E and D than today's youngsters.

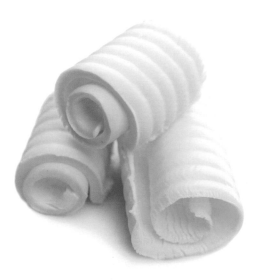

This, plus the low levels of pesticides, other chemicals and antibiotics in that earlier environment, must surely have provided protection against asthma.

An article in a recent *Courier Mail* claimed a study published in the July 2001 international journal, *Thorax*, found 'children who eat high quantities of margarine and vegetable oils may double their risk of asthma.' The study was of families living in the Lismore and Wagga Wagga areas of New South Wales, Australia.

Because of their high margarine intake, the children in the above study probably ate little or no butter. If their diets contained few other dairy products, they could have low reserves of vitamin A thereby making them more prone to asthma.

Recently I saw a newspaper advertisement for Shark Liver Oil for children. (I'm not criticising shark liver oil – I know nothing about it.) I was upset however to see the advertisers proudly stating their product was low in vitamins A and D – **only** 25 units! As if it was something to boast about!

At 25 units, a child could take a capsule each day for a month, and still not receive the vitamin A available from a good-sized carrot! While leafing through Lady Cilento's book *Medical Mother*, a paragraph seemed to leap from the page. It shows that vitamin A is beneficial in asthma, not only because it assists the adrenal glands to produce adrenaline and cortisone, but because it maintains the cells in the lungs. She wrote:

'When Vitamin A is deficient the surface cells die and all the respiratory tract, the nasal sinuses, Eustachian tubes to the ears, the lungs and smaller bronchial tubes become clogged with the desquamated dead cells, forming an excellent soil for the growth of bacteria and viruses of all kinds. The mucus, which is normally hostile to germs, is produced in abundance by the inflamed cells in an effort to cut off the infection....'

Many children and adults today, I believe, suffer from this simple deficiency.

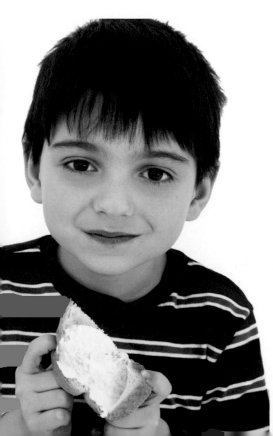

Polar bear liver and vitamin A overdose

It was exceptionally cold in Brisbane in 1990. Temperatures of one degree were recorded. As previously mentioned, cold weather triggers my asthma. Each day, I 'insured' against attacks by taking vitamins A, E and C to their limit (e.g. 60,000 units Vitamin A, 500mg Vitamin E, 3 teaspoons Vitamin C powder). On a couple of extremely cold days asthma forced me to increase the A to 80,000 units. Notwithstanding, it was a very successful year, asthma-wise.

There was one major incident, however, which I'm ashamed to admit. How many times had I heard the medical opinion regarding vitamin A and the dangers of overdose? So many times the following had been related to me: 'A group of explorers went to the Arctic where they ate nothing but polar-bear liver. These men subsequently died because polar bear liver is extremely high in vitamin A.'

On first hearing the polar bear story, I had difficulty maintaining a straight face. (First, catch your bear ...) We'd recently arrived home from a holiday in Sydney, where we'd searched Taronga Park Zoo and failed to find even one polar bear — maybe they'd eaten too many 'toxic' explorers.

This is not to say that too much vitamin A is not harmful. It certainly is, but then practically anything in overdose is harmful, even water. (Three deaths from water overdose were recorded by psychiatrists at the University of British Columbia.) A common English description for vitamin A overdose, is 'vitamin A intoxication'. A 'hangover' would be a more accurate description than 'intoxication'.

As implied earlier, during that winter in 1990, I accidentally overdosed on vitamin A.

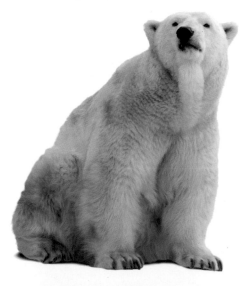

Looking back, I can't believe I did it. For some reason (probably economical) I bought some liquid vitamin A.

Somehow, after reading the instructions on the bottle, I believed that to obtain 10,000 units I had to fill the dropper completely instead of only to the indicating line.

This monumental mistake meant a dose of three to four times my usual cold weather amount, and the multiplication would have equaled approximately 250,000 units per day.

Why didn't I know something was wrong? Even when the drops were added to fruit juice, the taste was worse than dreadful. I knew I couldn't continue for long.

On the first night, I went to bed with a severe headache and took two aspirin — got that dose right. The second night, the same thing. The third night, ditto. I'm one of those lucky people who almost never suffers from headaches, so I knew something was wrong. At 2am the next night, the penny dropped. I remembered a wise woman's warning: 'You'll know if you ever overdose. The symptom is a severe headache.'

I jumped out of bed; the temperature was a freezing two degrees ('freezing' to Queenslanders anyway) and ran into the kitchen to re- read the label on the bottle. Sure enough I'd overdosed. No wonder my head was thumping. Within a day of ceasing all vitamin A, the headache disappeared.

I took no vitamins at all for the following week to allow my system to use up the excess. Neither my asthma nor general health suffered any ill effects from this overdose, although ever since that episode I can't bear the thought of liquid vitamin A!

It's not easy to overdose — but it can be done!

Looking back, I shouldn't take all the responsibility. Perhaps, I'm looking for an excuse but the instructions on the label were in very small print, and not very clear anyway. If I could make a mistake, surely others could do the same. Even when I understood the directions, the hand-eye co-ordination required to fill that darned dropper 'exactly to the line', was beyond.

It is not logical to label any substance 'dangerous' or 'poisonous' simply because it's possible to overdose on it. If this were so, all the following substances would have to be labeled 'POISON': tea, coffee, wine, spirits, aspirin etc, and as I said previously, even water.

Practically every 'good thing' can be overdone to the point where it becomes a 'bad thing'. It is my conviction that no-one, particularly asthmatics, should deny themselves adequate doses of vitamin A simply because it's possible to overdose.

Actually after my experience with vitamin A overdose, I'm amazed that anyone could continue long enough to arrive at the hair-loss and flaky-skin stage. The headaches would force most people to quit.

Some doctors persist in attacking vitamins A and E. Newspaper articles still appear from time to time showing bias against these vitamins, yet you don't often read about the dangers inherent in overdosing on *other* vitamins and minerals. My nutritionist claims it is possible to experience overdose symptoms on practically all of them. As Lady Cilento said 'the symptoms completely disappear in a few days after ceasing vitamin A'. (*Vitamin and Mineral Deficiencies* p.9.)

So why all the fuss?

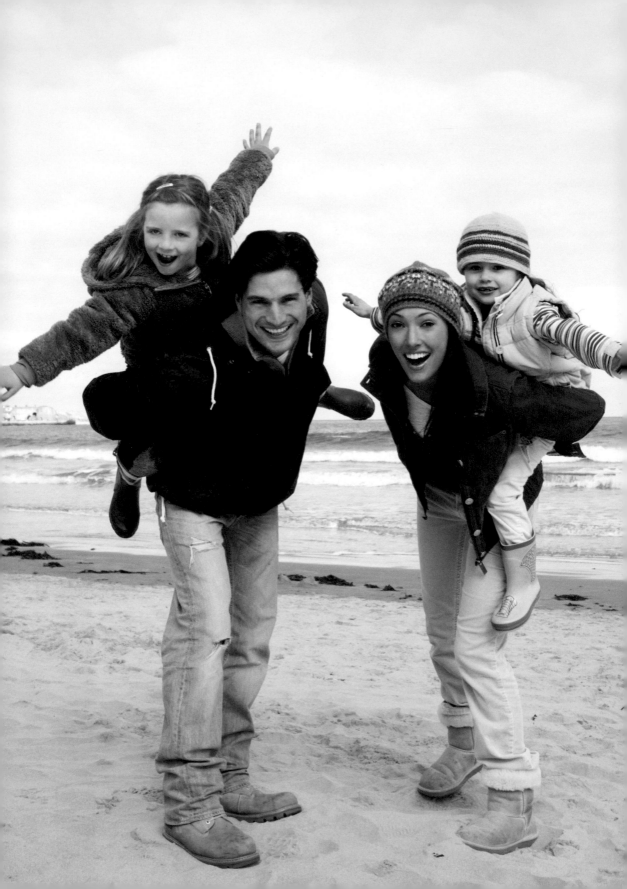

Watch for changes in the weather

Two things can have an unexpected effect on this vitamin treatment. One is change in the weather, particularly sudden drops in temperature and the other is ascertaining the correct type and dose of vitamin E. As previously stated, vitamin E is an essential ingredient in this treatment and ascertaining the correct amount of E is important.

I once saw some Accomin® Multi Vitamin Capsules, and noticed they contained 10,000 units of vitamin A, and 5 units of vitamin E. I decided they might be preferable to separate A and E capsules. Wrong! My chest tightened within two days of commencing them. Evidently **a good dose of Vitamin E** is required to make the treatment effective.

While on 10,000 units of vitamin A, I found 100mg of synthetic E was the minimum amount required to obtain results.

Synthetic E is very difficult to find these days, so I now use natural vitamin E and obtain it direct from the distributor. It has been successful, which no doubt means their product is fresh. The reason I rejected it in the first place was because it simply didn't work. However, I quote Dr M. Colgan's opinion on natural vitamin E:

'Buy it fresh. Vitamin E starts to oxidise in the capsules within a few months of manufacture.'

Dr Colgan also states:

'This is the one case where a natural vitamin is better than the synthetic.'
(From *Your Personal Vitamin Profile*, p. 147).

In the past, I may have bought stale natural vitamin E and that could have rendered it ineffective.

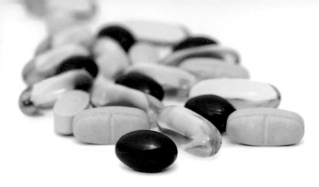

Another point which Lady Cilento stressed when speaking of fat soluble vitamins, is that they should be consumed with a meal containing a little fat or oil to call forth bile for their digestion.

As for the timing of vitamin doses, experience has taught me the most important dose of the day is at breakfast. Lunch and tea-time doses can be late, but in very cold weather, my 'preventative' breakfast dose must be taken before 9am.

The reason this first dose is important is that all my severe asthma attacks occurred at 3am or 4am. Research on rats has shown that vitamin A causes a 'beneficial compound to be formed in the lungs within 18 hours. (*Improving Your Health with Vitamin A*, p.15). I have also found through experience that there is about a twenty-hour time lapse before vitamin A begins to work. Therefore I have to ensure that the breakfast dose is taken so I will be protected in the early hours of the morning. To maintain good health, this timing is crucial for me during periods of infection or very cold weather.

Which brings me to another aspect of weather conditions. It is necessary to be conscious of uncharacteristic changes in temperatures.

Should the climate suddenly cool during the warmer months, vitamin A has to be increased — and **quickly**. Similarly a warm period during winter months, calls for a reduction in dose.

An example of a sudden drop in temperature happened in the winter of 1991 when I had to increase my vitamin A intake to 120,000 units for the short period of a week. (Don't faint I'm still alive and kicking.) The cold weather brought with it asthma.

Only large doses of A would control it. The remainder of winter was extremely mild and 40,000 units per day was sufficient.

You will probably consider 120,000 units a ridiculous amount of vitamin A, even for such a short period, but I need to prove that vitamin therapy is the complete answer, so I try to avoid all drugs. I would also ask you to remember that hormonal changes can exacerbate asthma. In the past I controlled it beautifully, for seven years, on very low doses of vitamin A. It is also worth remembering that (during those seven years) my son Danny and I required no medication, no special diet, no exercises, no meditation and very little faith — only the vitamins.

My advice to anyone harbouring doubts about vitamin treatment is simply this: 'Try it yourself for one week only and see how you feel.'

I'm convinced there is some psychological aspect to achieving the correct dose. I always get to the point where I don't want to increase the A, but when I remember the original premise Asthma is a Vitamin A Deficiency and I listen to my body's signals, I can happily take that little bit extra to make the symptoms disappear.

When we consider that, in times of crises, the amount of Ventolin® (administered by nebuliser) is multiplied by fifty and in some cases to the unbelievable amount of one hundred times, it is understandable why sufferers using only vitamins will sometimes need to substantially increase their usual dose. I have found during times of infections, etcetera it helps to abandon all fears of overdosing. Let's face it, vitamins can't possibly cause the over-dosing problems related to drugs, and what alternative is there? (To my mind, cortisone is not a viable alternative.)

These days I find myself saying, 'If I need it — I'll take it. If I don't — I won't.'

This table sets out my vitamin dosages over the years:

Age	Summer	Winter
38	Nil to 10,000 units vit.A, 100 mg. vit. E	10,000 to 20,000 i.u. vit.A, 100 mg. vit. E
43	10,000 i.u. vit. A 200 mg. vit. E	30,000 i.u. vit. A 400 mg. vit. E

Also started to add vitamin C powder for viruses.

Age	Summer	Winter
45-51	10,000 to 20,000 units vit.A, 200mg vit. E	60,000 i.u. vit. A 500mg vit. E 3 teasp. vit. C powder per day (if necessary)
53	10,000 to 20,000 500 i.u. vit. A i.u.natural vit. E	10,000 to 40,000 i.u. vit.A, 500 i.u. natural vit.E, 1 teasp. vit. C powder (Calc.Ascorbate)

After turning 53, my vitamin A requirement dropped, but now at 71, it has risen again to the previous age 45 level.

Dosage and deficiency dilemma

In order to keep bronchitis at bay while pregnant with the twins, I took an occasional 5,000 unit capsule of vitamin A. Recently however, there has been much controversy about pregnancy and vitamin A.

In 1991, I found a book (Antia F.P. *Clinical Dietetics and Nutrition* Bombay; Oxford University Press 1989) which stated that doses exceeding 10,000 units of vitamin A per day, should not be given to pregnant women **who are suffering vitamin A deficiencies**.

10,000 units seems conservative when we consider that a woman eating one meal of liver could ingest approx. 50,000 units of vitamin A.

Our tall, slender twins were (and still are) extremely healthy people, yet on a recent purchase of vitamin A tablets (5,000 units), I found the following:

'WARNING: Taking more than half a tablet per day during pregnancy may cause birth defects.'

Ridiculous! Half a tablet would equal 2,500 units.

Absolutely stunned, I rang the vitamin company to make inquiries. I was told that government regulations in July 1993 dictated that vitamin A must be sold with the above warning. The reason for the restriction was the reported fetal abnormalities produced by mothers ingesting 250,000 units of vitamin A per day.

Surely nobody could take 250,000 units for longer than a few days? Remember this was the toxic dose I accidentally took for three days. How could these women tolerate the headaches?

I've recently spoken to a few Health Department officials about this regulation and each time a different amount of vitamin A has been mentioned regarding the overdosing mothers. I've tried to get more information from Canberra but so far nothing has arrived.

A vitamin company representative said the regulation was an over- kill. What an understatement!

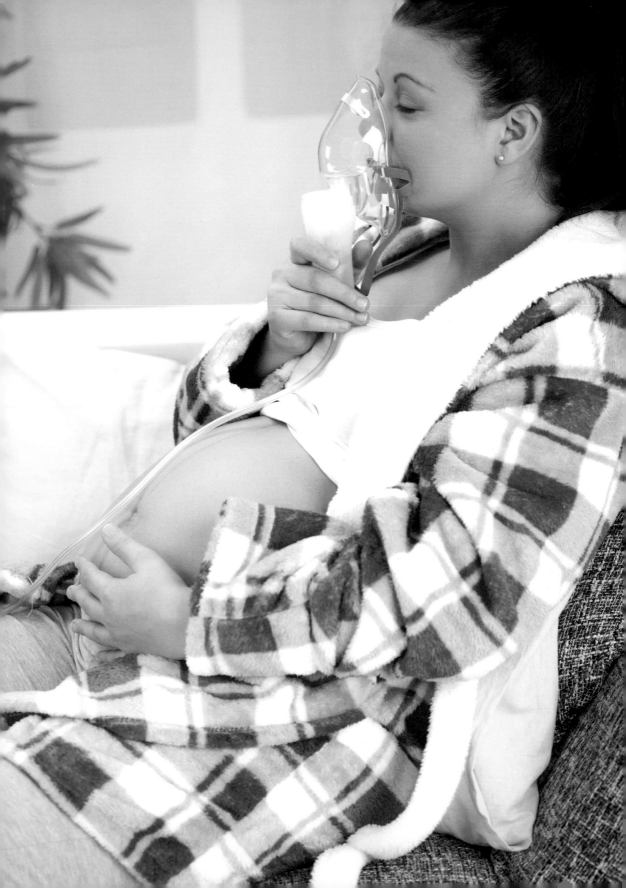

The Medical Journal of Australia Vol. 157, states that a South Australian report estimated the daily intake of vitamin A in that state to be 5,000 units. United States surveys show considerably higher averages of 7,000 - 8,000 i.u. per day.

Theoretically if 'more than 2,500 units per day may cause birth defects', South Australia and the United States of America should have very high incidences of birth defects, which of course is nonsense.

Pregnant women who suffer asthma must feel they are in a no-win situation. They are warned off vitamin A in doses higher than half a tablet, and yet medical information from MIMS (Intercontinental Medical Statistics) shows that the following drugs are not recommended during pregnancy:

• VENTOLIN®: Not to be used in pregnancy or if wanting to become pregnant. Drug passes over to baby. Not recommended for breastfeeding mothers.
• ORAL CORTICOSTEROIDS: In animal tests, these drugs produce abortion, cleft palate and skeletal malformations. Could reduce the performance of the adrenal glands in babies. Breastfeeding: Appears in breast-milk and could suppress growth of baby or reduce functions of adrenal glands.
POISON S4
• NUELIN®: Appears in breast milk so doses must be kept low to avoid toxicity to baby.

If doctors are concerned that too much vitamin A harms the foetus, shouldn't they also be concerned about medication transferring to the baby?

Where are the WARNINGS on Cortisone, Ventolin® or Nuelin® labels?

Is the government relying on doctors to warn women? Can all doctors remember to warn **every** woman of child-bearing age of the dangers of cortisone and other drugs?

Do they ask if she is breast-feeding? Would they know she is **thinking** of becoming pregnant? The warnings should be clearly printed on the labels.

The same nutrition book which espouses conservative doses of vitamin A in pregnancy, goes on to state that where severe deficiencies are common, such as in India, women are given a dose of 200,000 units of vitamin A immediately following delivery of their babies. This is to build up the A in the mother's milk supply. Evidently milk must not deliver too much vitamin A to the baby.

There certainly seems to be confusion regarding pregnancy and vitamin A. Doctor Antia writes that numerous babies and children in India suffer blindness because of vitamin A deficiencies (even well-off children) yet, in Australia, doctors warn pregnant women off vitamin A completely.

Lady Cilento claimed foetal abnormalities are caused by a lack of vitamin A and the book *Biochemical Basis of Medicine* 1985, backs up her claim with a list of nine symptoms of vitamin A deficiency.

A precis of that list includes the following symptoms: Inability to see in the dark; failure of growth; dryness of mucus membranes of lungs, digestive tract, urinary tract and secondary infection; faulty bone modelling; nerve lesions; abnormal enlargement of the head; **degeneration of testes and abortion or production of malformed offspring**; certain forms of skin disease; death (resulting from serious deficiency).

The book then proceeds to list six symptoms of vitamin A overdose: Failure of growth (rat); skin abnormalities (rat and man); increased pressure in skull (infant); vomiting (man); bone abnormalities (man); fatal internal hemorrhage (rat); birth malformations (rat).

An interesting point here is that these overdose symptoms are similar to the deficiency symptoms.

Is this indicating that a pregnant woman with too little vitamin A in her system risks miscarriage or malformed offspring and one who is overdosing runs the same risk?

Personally, I would be much more concerned about too little vitamin A than too much. Australians on the whole would be more likely to be deficient in this vitamin. Lady Cilento said that from her observations of ordinary diets, she found many to be 'woefully deficient' in vitamin A. (*Medical Mother* p.86).

Let us consider an average nourishing Australian meal consisting of roast chicken, white potatoes, corn on the cob and cabbage followed by a plate of fresh peaches and ice-cream (not homemade). First class meal, we would say, but that meal would deliver only a fraction of the 1985 Recommended Daily Allowance of 5,000 units of vitamin A.

Unless a pregnant woman made up the shortfall in the remaining meals or ate one liver meal during the week, she would be deficient according to these standards. As excess vitamin A is stored in the body, one large meal of liver should supply the minimum requirements of vitamin A for a week, but we must bear in mind that some people have difficulty extracting fat-soluble vitamins from their food, plus there is the likelihood of high pesticide levels in the liver meal.

If I were young, pregnant and asthmatic, I would aim for the middle ground and follow Lady Cilento's advice by ensuring my diet contained sufficient vitamin A foods. I would also add 10,000 units of vitamin A, plus about 250mg of vitamin E per day.

As previously mentioned, those occasional vitamin A capsules (5,000 units) during my pregnancy certainly did not harm the twins. As babies they possessed an extremely high resistance to infection and this resistance continued throughout kindergarten, school and even university.

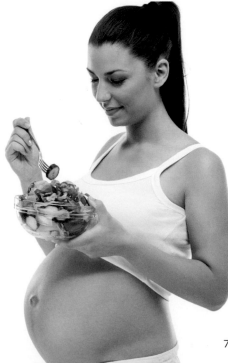

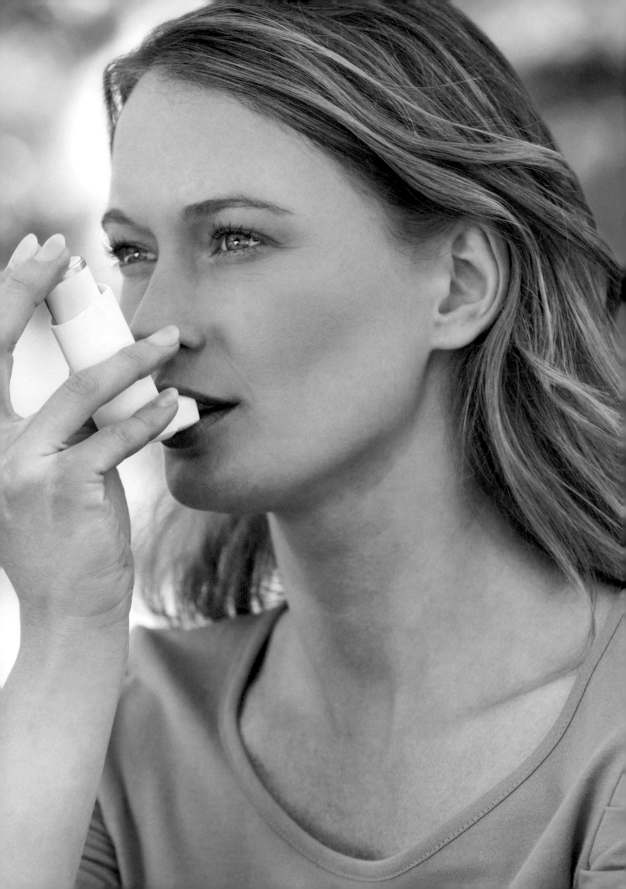

How safe are our asthma drugs?

New Zealand, like Australia, experienced dramatic increases in asthma deaths after 1965 and Fenoterol was linked with this increased death rate. A spokesman for the Wellington School of Medicine said:

'While modern methods for treating asthma have improved the quality of life of many asthmatics, mortality has continually increased during the period of their introduction and use.'

In May 1989, the New Zealand Health Department advised doctors treating severe asthmatics, to use alternatives to Fenoterol.

To my knowledge, Fenoterol is not widely used in Australia. Salbutamol (Ventolin®), however, a similar (but weaker) drug is freely used here and is also suspect. Why Ventolin® earned disrepute has not been fully explained. Suddenly we are being told the largest selling asthma drug in Australia could be dangerous with long-term use. Why are we not being told the full story on Ventolin®? Surely simply stating 'it could be dangerous' is not enough?

If Ventolin® puffers are hazardous, what does this make Ventolin® delivered by nebuliser? The dose received by this method is medically estimated to be fifty times that of the puffer.

At an asthma seminar in 1984 attended by world leaders in asthma research, one doctor claimed:

'What I am convinced about, as has been shown in the majority of studies of patients with asthma, is that conventional doses of beta-adrenoceptor agonists do not cause development of tolerance or resistance. I think it is important to state that this applies to conventional doses, but may not be true for nebulised doses. We are studying long term use in nebulisers, where there is a suggestion that there is development of resistance.'

A further claim by a second doctor is as follows:

'My feeling is that asthmatics are in an unusual position, in that they are given these inhalers to use according to subjective symptoms that they experience; when they do not have relief they get scared and take more of the drug, so it is all very well to say that, under very controlled conditions, they take this dose regularly at such and such a time and you can set up studies to prove that, but, one can never be sure that that is the way that asthmatics use their medihalers. There is a very real possibility that at least a group of these people over use such medication and induce tachyphylaxis.'

The first doctor responded:

'In Britain, patients tend to underuse rather than overuse their inhaler, because there has been concern about overusing inhalers, and the dose that is recommended is quite small, so I think that it must be a very small minority who actually really overuse their inhalers. I think that the problem is with nebulisers where the dose is about fifty fold greater and it may be that people are using much larger doses there.'

A third doctor interjected with:

'The really large doses of beta-adrenoceptor agonists (Berotec®, Ventolin®, Bricanyl® etc.) are given when people come into hospital with bad asthma.'

As we can see, doubts regarding bronchodilators (Ventolin® etc.) were being expressed by these experts as far back as 1984.

Further interesting information came from a fourth doctor/ researcher, who said:

'I remember a case report in the literature on cod-liver oil and asthma, and I think it was referred to in a lecture of Professor Burn some time ago, implying that cod-liver oil was very good in asthmatic diseases. Do you think we have to consider dietary modification of fluidity in membranes as a potentially effective therapy in asthmatic diseases?'

A fifth added:

'That is a difficult question. A couple of years ago, I was on an ad hoc committee of life sciences, to deliberate on how the diet can influence such function. It was concluded that there was no concrete evidence for this type of suggestion.'

A sixth man finalised the discussion with the comment:

'It is interesting that, when you let the discussion run, eventually the nutritional question does emerge and it is obviously an appropriate time for lunch.'

Note: the first doctor said that some asthmatics may overuse their bronchodilating inhalers and induce 'tachyphylaxis.' To most of us, this word sounds positively awesome. But according to the medical dictionary 'tachyphylaxis' means: 'Rapidly decreasing response to a drug or physiologically active agent after a few doses.'

This definition (containing the words **rapidly** and **few**) is extremely worrying. Even today some asthma sufferers are instructed to use bronchodilators four times daily.

In a letter to the editor of *The Courier Mail* in October 1990, a vice patron of the Asthma Foundation stated he had received a telex from a drug company which manufactures bronchodilators. This company claimed two world asthma authorities, who previously warned against long-term use of bronchodilators, have since changed their commentary to read as follows:

'There is no doubt about the safety of asthma relieving drugs such as Ventolin®, Bricanyl®, Berotec® and Raspolin® — all bronchodilators.'

The vice patron expressed amazement that this turn-about should occur, considering that Berotec® (Fenoterol) had been incriminated in the increased mortality rate in New Zealand.

It would seem likely that should there be any concerns about drug tolerance, or overdose reactions from bronchodilators, Queensland would have more problems than, say, England. In 1995 it seemed every second asthmatic in Queensland owned or rented a nebuliser. I heard a young mother at an asthma lecture say, 'The kindergarten my child attends has refused to continue attaching children to their nebulisers during the lunch hour, because those without asthma are being neglected.'

An elderly pensioner rang a Brisbane Open Line radio station to say he required seven or eight asthma prescriptions per week. Another woman rang to say a friend of hers had three children on full-time asthma medication.

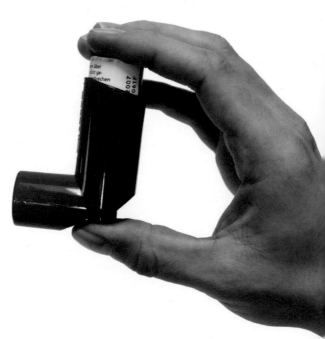

An extract from a letter to the magazine *Breathing Space*, January 1987, outlines the regime maintained by a young woman:

- 2 x 250 SR Nuelin® 3 times a day
- Ventolin® 3 x day - 2 puffs
- Becloforte® 3 x day - 2 puffs
- Nebuliser 3 x day
- Bricanyl® 7.5mg - 1 at night

Six Nuelin® a day seems incredible to one who gets the jitters from only one tablet. The whole thing is mind-boggling. In my opinion there's no wonder this person is ill! The nonchalance some asthma sufferers use inhaled bronchodilators indicates these medications are often regarded as harmless. A secondary school teacher told me he knew of instances where students handed puffers around the entire class. He said they got a 'high' from the puffers.

I wonder if people who abuse bronchodilators connect their headaches, irritability, rapid heart rate and skeletal muscle tremor, with the over-use of their puffer? MIMS (Intercontinental Medical Statistics) states that nebulisers can cause potentially serious disturbance of heart rhythm plus possible heart muscle damage with high dosage over long periods.

These are not minor dangers. The cost to Australia in supplying medication for such a large number of asthma sufferers is astronomical. The total combined cost to the Federal and State Governments as listed by the National Asthma Campaign in 1991, amounted to 329 million dollars. One wonders how long governments can continue subsidising such amounts. More to the point, I wonder what period the body can continue absorbing such high levels of drugs before damage occurs.

Australians do not appear to share the British fear of inhalers. Actually Australia and New Zealand has a much higher death rate from asthma than England. In 1981, England had a mortality rate (ages 5 - 34 years) of almost 1 per 100,000 of population. (From *Asthma — Its Management In General Practice*). Australia with 538 deaths in 1981 had approximately **3 per 100,000**. In 1987 with 803 deaths, this Australian mortality rate had risen to approximately **5 per 100,000**. This is shocking, particularly when countries such as Scandinavia and America, like Britain, have low mortality rates.

Thankfully Australia has since experienced a huge reduction in the mortality rate, with the number falling to 314 in the year 2003. This is wonderful, however, according to a report by the Australian Centre for Asthma Monitoring in August 2005, we still suffer asthma at high levels compared to international standards, with one in seven children and one in nine adults being diagnosed with this illness.

Another puzzling aspect is that England has had an increase in the overall numbers of asthmatics, whereas Denmark and Finland have not. What are the inhabitants of Denmark and Finland doing right? Thankfully, results of research published in *The Lancet* of December 1990 indicate a change in the use of bronchodilators is being considered:

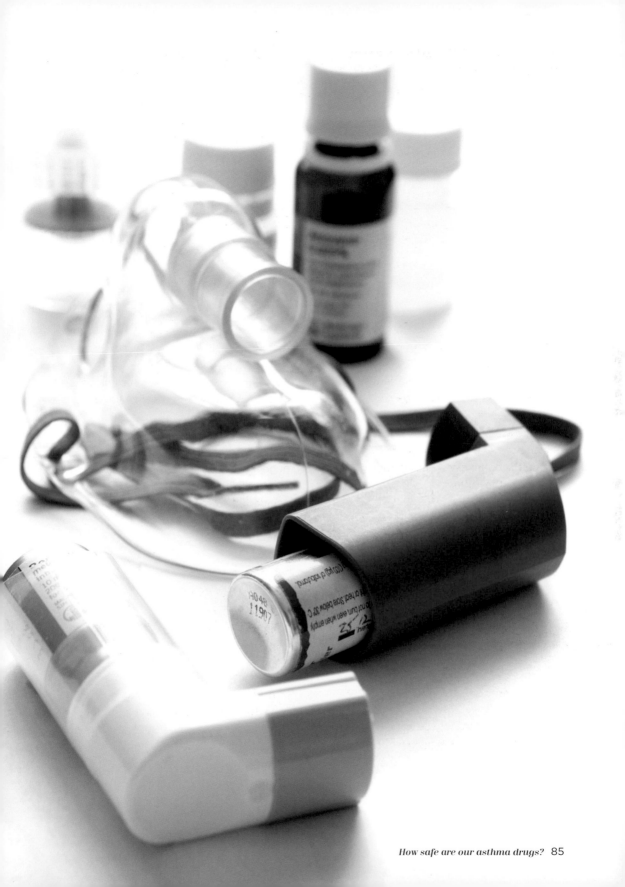

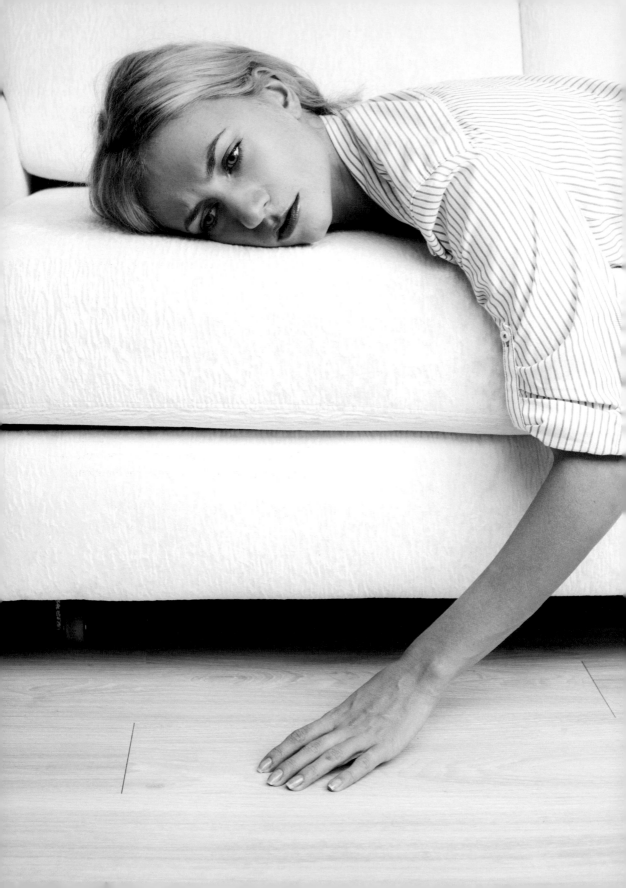

'A New Zealand study of 88 asthma patients found that only 30% improved when treated with regular doses of the inhaled bronchodilator, Fenoterol. Seventy percent improved when treated with the drug only at the time of an asthma attack.

The Lancet published an accompanying editorial criticising bronchodilators, and called on doctors and drug companies to re-define the use of such drugs in treatment.

Physicians who manage patients with asthma are therefore confronted with the uncomfortable possibility that a mainstay of treatment may be harmful, just when long acting (bronchodilators) are about to be introduced. Enthusiasm for such effective drugs will need to be tempered by the findings of the two new studies.'

Many people are also concerned about the use of oral **steroids** in asthma. On a visit to our State Library, I studied an edition of MIMS and found a list of side effects from the oral steroids used in the treatment of asthma. It was truly frightening!

I wondered whether those on oral steroids would connect symptoms such as insomnia and severe depression (sometimes bordering on psychotic) to these drugs.

I think the oral steroid side effects of cataracts and osteoporosis are commonly known, but what of others cited in MIMS, such as menstrual irregularities, moon face, personality changes, hypertension, peptic ulcer, low resistance to infection, congestive heart failure in susceptible patients and muscle weakness etcetera.

Added to this, is the concern that some may never be able to cease using steroids. I've heard of cases where adrenal glands stop functioning because a person has been on synthetic cortisone for too long. These people are then forced to take steroids for the rest of their lives.

Are you aware of these problems?

You might say, 'But what about the effects of vitamin A overdose?' Well yes, but they are reversible, and we are talking overdose. The adverse effects of steroids as mentioned in MIMS, occur with **normal** and long-term use of **prescribed** doses. Overdose is not mentioned.

As we know, medication is life saving on occasions, and **must** be on hand in case of emergency.

What is particularly worrying many asthmatics, however, is the sheer quantity they are told to administer. Surely our principal aim must be to reduce the number of drugs, while still maintaining a good quality of life.

It finally happened

I couldn't believe it! They had gone ahead and done it.

I received a notice from my vitamin distributor informing me that a government regulation passed in July 1993, forbid over-the-counter sale of any vitamin A exceeding 5,000 units. This vitamin company has ceased manufacturing 10,000 unit capsules. Phone calls to various other retailers brought the same response. I was told, however, that a Sydney company was still producing 9,000 unit tablets. I rang their pharmacist who informed me he was only permitted to sell to doctors, chemists, dentists and hospitals. 'If you want these capsules, you will need a doctor's prescription. It's absolutely ridiculous!' he said. 'This regulation should never have gone through. Our company fought it all on our own. Did you know that 10,000 unit capsules are now registered S4 on the Poisons Register?'

'They can't be!' I exclaimed. 'Only the other day I read that cortisone is marked POISON S4. How can vitamin A be the same?'
'You've got me. Are they going to make people get doctor's prescriptions now to go to the butcher, because 100g of liver contains 50,000 units of vitamin A?'

'I know — is Australia the only country doing this?

'Yes,' he replied, 'you can still buy them everywhere else.'

Following this conversation, I began to wonder, 'Who makes the decision that vitamin A and cortisone should both be classed Poison S4?'

I rang more pharmacists then, only to be told that even if I did have a doctor's prescription they would be unable to supply me with 10,000 unit capsules. They had none in stock. They could however, order some for me.

One chemist knew of two companies still selling 10,000 unit capsules. Unfortunately, the first brand, the one belonging to the chemist I spoke to in Sydney, contained fillers which upset my stomach, so that left only one company. Their capsules are based on soy-bean oil which I tolerate well and their headquarters are also in Sydney, so I rang their chemist who advised me: 'Stockpile while you can. We are ceasing the production of 10,000 unit capsules and at the end of the year we commence making only 2,500 unit doses. The authorities say we don't need any extra fat-soluble vitamins.'

'Well, what are people like me supposed to do?' I inquired, 'or aren't there many on the higher doses?'

'Actually,' he said, 'I've had quite a few calls like yours. One lady from Melbourne was absolutely frantic.'

'I can understand why. I'm beginning to think people like me can't absorb fat soluble vitamins from our food.'

'That's right,' he said, 'you probably lack the proper enzymes.'

'I suppose I'll have to send overseas when my stock-pile runs out then?'

'Yes.' he replied.

After some heavy ringing around, I managed to find three Australia-wide companies still selling 5,000 unit capsules. Unfortunately, one of the brands (the one most easily available) causes me severe abdominal distress. Still the other two types are agreeable. Asthmatics, therefore, requiring only moderate Vitamin A doses, should encounter few difficulties. If, however, the only available dose is 2,500 units, those over forty needing higher doses could be forced to take at least 16 capsules per day and perhaps 24 during mid-winter. This age group would have trouble swallowing not only the capsules but also the cost attached to this bureaucratic overkill.

America passed a law forbidding the labelling of vitamin A as poisonous. Australia must do likewise. (Registering vitamin A on the Poison's Register and marking it S4, certainly gives the impression that it is poisonous or at least dangerous.)

How can a product be 'safe' in one country and 'poisonous' in another?

Why is Australia so swift to restrict vitamin A when it is so disgracefully slow in following America's lead in banning dangerous pesticides? American experts believe many pesticides are carcinogenic. Vitamin A is considered by authorities such as Dr Michael B. Sporn, of the American National Cancer Institute, to be one of the chief nutrients in the battle against cancer — and it is allowed in America in strengths deemed 'poisonous' in Australia.

Madness!

Not long after these restrictions, I visited a huge chemist shop in the city and, out of curiosity, asked if they had any vitamin A. The shop assistant replied they didn't stock vitamin A anymore. 'It causes birth defects, you know.' (We can't blame the shop assistant for repeating what she'd been told, but it's worrying to think of the people she may have convinced.)

They did stock cod-liver oil capsules (5,000 i.u.vit.A) so I bought some and was staggered to read the following warning: 'Taking more than five-eighths of a capsule during pregnancy may cause birth defects.'

This is good old-fashioned cod-liver oil we're talking about. It's been around since Moses! By the way, how does one take five-eighths of a capsule?

Another shock awaited me on reading the labels on two well-known brands of multivitamin capsules. Neither contained any vitamin A (not even beta-carotene) and one brand even declared itself to be 'retinol free'.

NOTE: Retinol is the technical name for basic vitamin A.

It is advisable to read the contents listed on the label before buying multivitamins. You may not be getting any vitamin A at all.

As I still hadn't received any information from Canberra on why this new regulation had been passed, I decided to ring and make inquiries.

I had a lengthy conversation with a bureaucratic gentleman who told me the new regulation was not trying to frighten people off vitamin A and he was upset to hear of my experience in the large chemist shop. He said the regulation was brought in to protect the public from over-dosing, which was a concern in one of the states where there had been publicity about vitamin A preventing cancer. I told him I believed that could be true. He ignored my comment and said there was evidence that overdosing on vitamin A caused birth defects, and he would send me this information. As it transpired I waited nearly ten months.

Here we are, with thousands suffering cancer or asthma, plus umpteen people abusing drugs and all the authorities can do, is worry that someone might overdose on vitamin A! Shouldn't they be shouting from the rooftops, 'Hey, everyone, whatever you do, don't become deficient in vitamin A.'

While waiting for the information from Canberra, my daughter, Melissa, suggested that *The Medical Journal of Australia* might contain relevant information.

After searching through past copies of this journal at the State Library, I found and read an article in the December 1992 issue.

It was a lengthy report on the potential for birth defects of vitamin A, and its 'congeners'.

Speaking purely as a lay person there appeared to be sufficient proof to incriminate the drugs which are **synthetic derivatives** of vitamin A and used in the treatment of acne and psoriasis. However, from the evidence presented in this paper, I still cannot understand why **natural vitamin A** would be vilified.

Even after tracking back through medical journals to find the original source of this hysteria, I am still amazed that vitamin A should be so severely restricted. The original evidence appears to be pathetic. It consists of a list of 18 cases of birth abnormalities presented in a copy of the Rosa FW, Wilk AL, Kelsey FO, (1986) *Teratogen Update: Vitamin A Congeners* 'Teratology paper.

The 18 women listed in the case study gave birth to babies with abnormalities. They had been taking natural vitamin A.

Four of the 18 examples can be disregarded immediately as they were overdosing, (in some cases, grossly) and we have seen earlier that overdosing causes birth defects in rats.

One woman took 500,000 units during the first and second months. How could anyone survive a dose like that, even if it was only for a few days? (You really would have to wonder about this woman.) Another took 50,000 units of vitamin D. That would also be massive overdosing of that vitamin.

We are left with 14 cases on the list. One contains no dosage information at all, so it must be disregarded. Of the remaining 13 some were taking doses of 18,000+, some 25,000, some 40,000, some 50,000 and even 60,000 units daily, before and throughout their pregnancy.

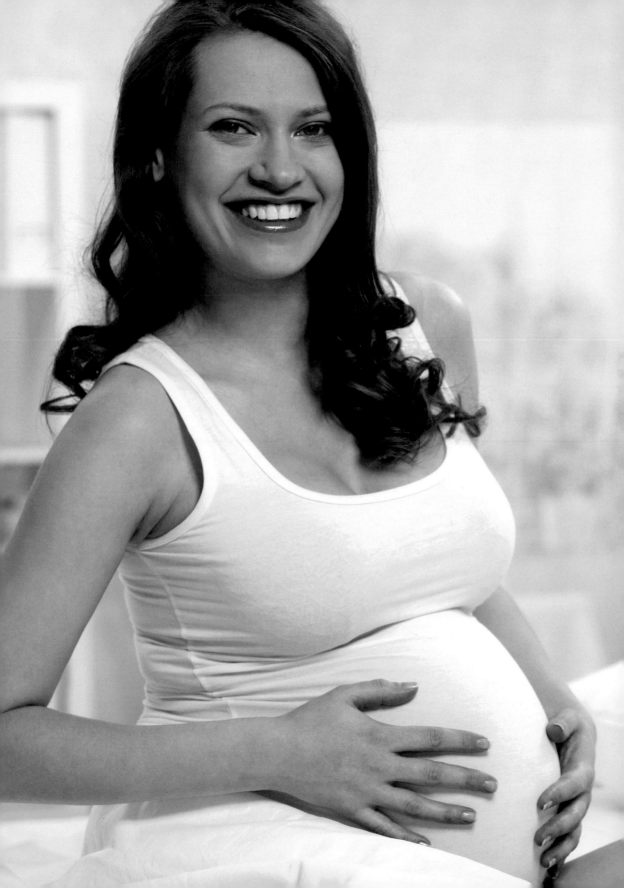

Why were these pregnant women taking such high doses of vitamin A? Their ages are not mentioned, but surely few would be over 40. In young women, most respiratory problems would, I'm sure, respond to much lower doses than those mentioned above.

The anomalies pertaining to these 13 cases are as follows:

(a) No data is supplied as to why these women were taking such high doses of vitamin A.

(b) Ages are not mentioned.

(c) No dates are recorded.

(d) No doctor or researcher's name is mentioned.

(e) Some don't even mention the country of origin.

They are so lacking in data that an analytical chemist said, 'Evidence like that would never stand up in a court of law.' No control studies have been carried out either, and the medical journal article added: 'At this time no denominators exist for developing control rates.'

I can't get any extra information on these cases because the details are not published in any scientific paper. They are only on this list which according to a spokesman from the State Library could have been a handout at a presentation.

I spoke to a pharmacist about the 18 birth defect cases. He too must have seen this paper, because he expressed surprise that vitamin A should have been considered responsible for the birth defects when there was no indication whether the mothers had been smoking marijuana or drinking excess alcohol during the pregnancies.

Canberra finally forwarded the promised 'evidence' of birth defects caused by vitamin A. Incredibly it was exactly the same 'list' which I'd previously found.

So! This is why pregnant women are warned off all sources of vitamin A in excess of 2,500 units.

If people like me don't come out and call this pathetic, who will?

Who cares enough about vitamin A to raise his/her voice?

Who has the right and the obligation to speak out?

Me, that's who!

There is an interesting section in the 1992 *Australian Medical Journal* article, which refers to cancer. I quote: '... an absence of retinoids (vitamin A) produces a deregulation of cell growth, similar to that seen in carcinogenesis (cancer).'

This quote is fascinating because my old book on vitamin A, published in 1978, said the same thing.

NOTE: The journal article used the word 'absence' not 'deficiency'.

Are the writers saying that cells containing no vitamin A look like cancer cells? Could it be they look like cancer cells, because they are cancer cells?

The Recommended Daily Allowance for vitamin A has also been changed. According to the 1980 American Chart shown earlier, a male adult and a pregnant woman both require a minimum 5,000 units of vitamin A per day. In 1994 the Australian Health department advised 'The recommended adult daily amount of vitamin A **from all sources** is 2,500 i.u.'

The wording 'from all sources' is amazing.

According to these new daily requirements, eating more than two eggs per day and a cheese sandwich, would be overdosing on vitamin A and if pregnant could cause birth defects!

Someone has it wrong. Very soon, only 2,500 unit capsules will be in our shops. When this happens, theoretically, we should not only require a doctor's prescription to purchase liver, we should also need one for carrots or spinach.

More madness!

We can't survive without vitamin A, so why are the powers-that-be trying so hard to scare everyone off it?

I ask, 'Is vitamin A seen as a threat to drug companies?'

Each day new evidence appears on the adverse effects of asthma medication and the benefits of vitamin A for various cancers, then suddenly only very low doses of this vitamin are available. Is this a coincidence?

While speaking with doctors and chemists, I am continually amazed that they are only interested in the dangers of vitamin A overdose. Very few have been impressed by the fact that I've been free of asthma for 33 years.

Soon there will be no point paying money to wheedle a prescription from a doctor, because higher doses of this vitamin will not be available. Hopefully, the three companies mentioned earlier, will continue producing 5,000 unit capsules. I predict that the new 2,500 unit doses will cost almost as much as the old 10,000 unit capsules.

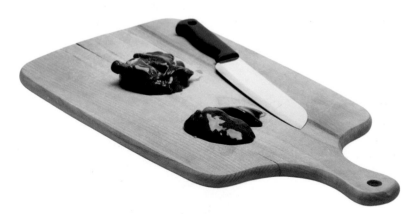

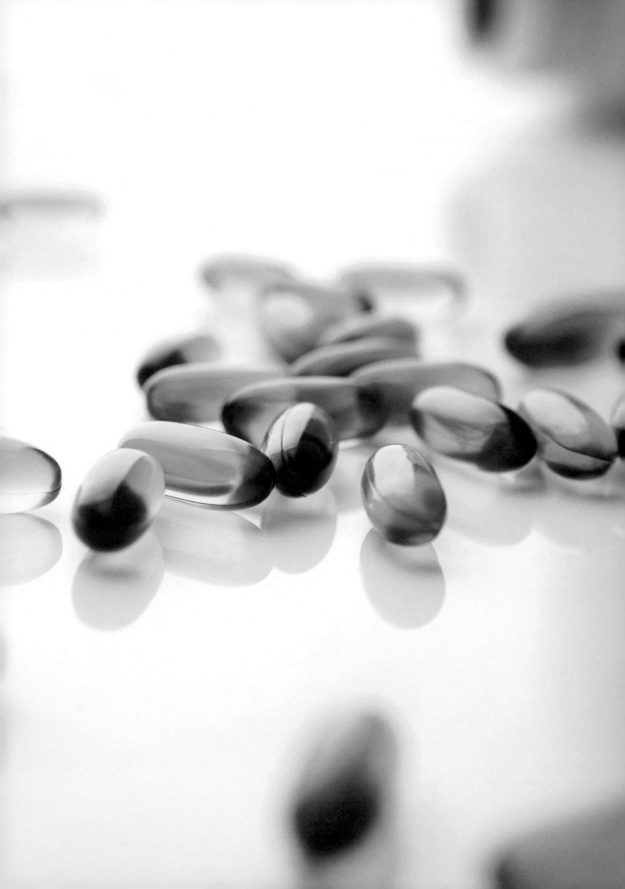

Cod-liver oil or A+D wouldn't be suitable for people like me who take high dosages — we'd soon overdose on vitamin D.

NOTE: Bio Concepts, Kelvin Grove, Queensland states that doses of Vitamin D, in excess of 4,000 units per day, constitute an overdose.

Beta-carotene, of which only one sixth converts to vitamin A, would be useless. My nutritionist said, 'Only straight vitamin A would work for you, Marian.' I'm sure I couldn't stomach lamb's fry every day and diabetics who cannot convert carotene into vitamin A may also have problems.

If I have to choose between those who parrot current scare-tactics and the teachings of esteemed doctors, I will follow Doctors Pauling, Sporn, and Lady Cilento every time.

When it comes to asthma, I've proven Lady Cilento's teachings are true. Whatever would she say if she were alive today?

This regulation is ridiculous. If vitamin A is 'poisonous', why don't we need a doctor's prescription to purchase whisky? Being treated like an idiot infuriates me; 10,000 unit capsules should be freely available and mothers must not be told moderate amounts of vitamin A cause birth defects.

Let the madness cease.

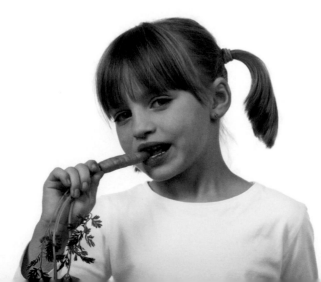

Phenomenal Fall in Childhood Asthma

The outlook for asthmatics is improving all the time. The most stunning news is the reduction in childhood asthma rates, which in many places seems to have dropped more than half over the past 10 years. The latest figures show as few as 9.9% of children now suffer from asthma. During the 1970s, 80s and 90s, we were told constantly that the childhood asthma rate was 20% to 25%.

The doctor announcing the new figure of 9.9% said he didn't know what had brought about this halving of the childhood rate.

I first became aware of the fall in numbers in 2010 when a middle aged teacher in Brisbane asked me if I knew why so few children these days suffered from asthma. She said there was a noticeable improvement since her earlier teaching days.

Following the latest Institute Of Health and Welfare report, I contacted primary schools and heard a similar story. A spokeswoman from a school at Mt. Gravatt, Queensland, said, 'We have 375 children at the school and 23 are asthmatic, so that means 6% have asthma'. Another local primary school here in Newcastle with an enrolment of 300 reported 20 asthma sufferers. This is around 7%.

What has happened? Does anyone know? These numbers are phenomenal. As mentioned later in this book, when my daughters were in primary school, there were five or six asthmatics in each class! Something has definitely changed and so far we've been given no public explanation for this turn around.

On examining reports from the Australian Bureau of Statistics, it appears asthma in children has been declining gradually over recent years. In 2005 it was recorded at 12%.

I rang the Asthma Foundation and was told the latest childhood rate of 9.9% just **appears** very low because the previous rate was artificially high. They also told me children under five were not counted.

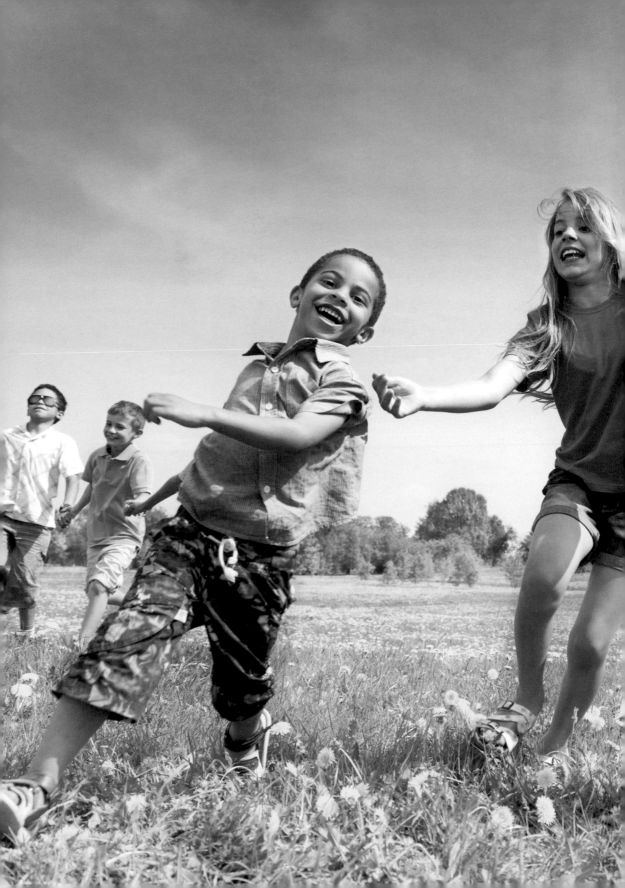

This explanation for the fall in numbers is **not** very convincing. I believe the percentage ten years ago was correct and not artificially high. As mentioned earlier, the rate of asthma in children has been elevated for several decades, not just 10 years ago. And as for not recording children under five, the 2012 graph from the Bureau of Statistics – 'Profiles of Health, 2011-13' includes children from 0 to 14 years and reports their rate at 11.4% for males and 7.2% for females. This equates to the above level of 9.9%.

Even if those under five were not included, surely that wouldn't make such a huge difference to the statistics as these children are often diagnosed with asthmatic bronchitis (as my son was at four years of age), croup or some other childhood bronchial problem.

There could be many reasons for this reduction, but naturally I like to think mothers now believe asthma is a vitamin A deficiency and give their susceptible children vitamins A and E!

Or alternatively, perhaps the improvement connects to the addition of vitamin A to margarine. This occurred by law in 1987. Prior to the late 1960s, few people ate margarine, as it was white in colour and had an unappetising appearance. In Australia, colouring was not allowed in margarine until 1960. Butter, which naturally contains vitamin A, was the preferred spread. But after 1970, most consumers switched to margarine because of the scare campaigns against butter and dairy products.

Therefore since margarine at that time had no vitamin A, and butter was considered unacceptable, the population missed a vital source of fat soluble vitamin A for twenty years.

According to Wikipedia, in 1940 many European countries made adding vitamin A to margarine compulsory because of the advent of war. Fresh butter was difficult to obtain and had to be transported from Australia and New Zealand. Due to the frequency of submarine attacks, little butter arrived. The fact that most Europeans received this additional vitamin A for over seventy years, might explain the low asthma death rate in those countries.

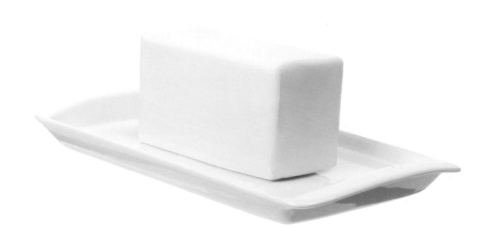

America has also enjoyed low death rates for many decades. I've not been able to ascertain just when vitamin A was first added to margarine in America, but by law there has to be 15,000 i.u. of vitamin A per pound (about 500g) of margarine and Vitamin D is optional in that country (from the FDA USA website). Australia now requires a similar amount of vitamin A to be added to margarine.

In England, a recent reduction in asthma among all ages has been linked to restrictions placed on smoking in public. At first glance we might think this could also apply to Australia, but we have to remember the smoking rate for men in the 1950s and 1960s was very high yet asthma in children was rare. Women, on the other hand, smoked very little until around the early 1970s.

Our fourth child was born in 1973 and while in hospital my room-mate and I were astonished to see smoke billowing from the open door of the maternity ward across the hall. This ward had empty ice-cream tins at the foot of each bed for the collection of cigarette butts. Could this have anything to do with the sudden increase in childhood asthma? Could maternal smoking cause asthma when paternal smoking did not?

Of course, these days, there's also more attention given to foods that might induce asthma. That awareness has no doubt brought about a reduction in some children.

Considering these various hypotheses, the one I believe most likely to have produced the most widespread improvement, is the addition of vitamin A to margarine. So many children eat margarine and only something so widely used could result in this dramatic change. Very low doses of vitamins are needed to prevent a deficiency disease. For instance, we need only

tiny amounts of vitamin C to prevent scurvy yet once the illness has manifested, larger doses are required to reverse it.

Perhaps it's the same with asthma. Many small children might never develop asthma today because vitamin A is added to margarine; and because they receive this small dose constantly, they may be protected throughout their childhood.

I'm no expert on this, and I know it's important scientifically not to jump to conclusions, but until I hear a more persuasive theory, I'm holding firm to this one.

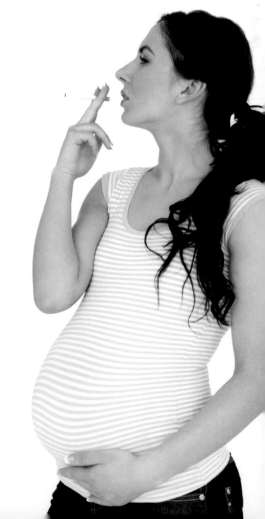

Exciting Research from Japan

Some important research has been undertaken in Japan. In 2006, a group of doctors from the Department of Pediatrics, Jikei University School of Medicine, Tokyo, tested well-nourished asthmatic children in Japan to evaluate their levels of vitamin A and E.

The authors found the 'vitamin A concentrations were significantly lower in asthmatic children than controls' (which would have been non-asthmatic children). I won't list the whole confusing analysis, except to say the asthmatic children recorded 19.41 of vitamin A concentration compared to the healthy children who had 29.52.

They concluded the data suggested 'there is a correlation between vitamin A deficiency and the mechanism of asthmatic response' They went on to say the data supports the theory that low levels of vitamin A affect both the acute response and the chronic damage of airways.

Exciting stuff! Here's hoping this research gets a lot of publicity. (Although we haven't heard much about it so far, have we?)

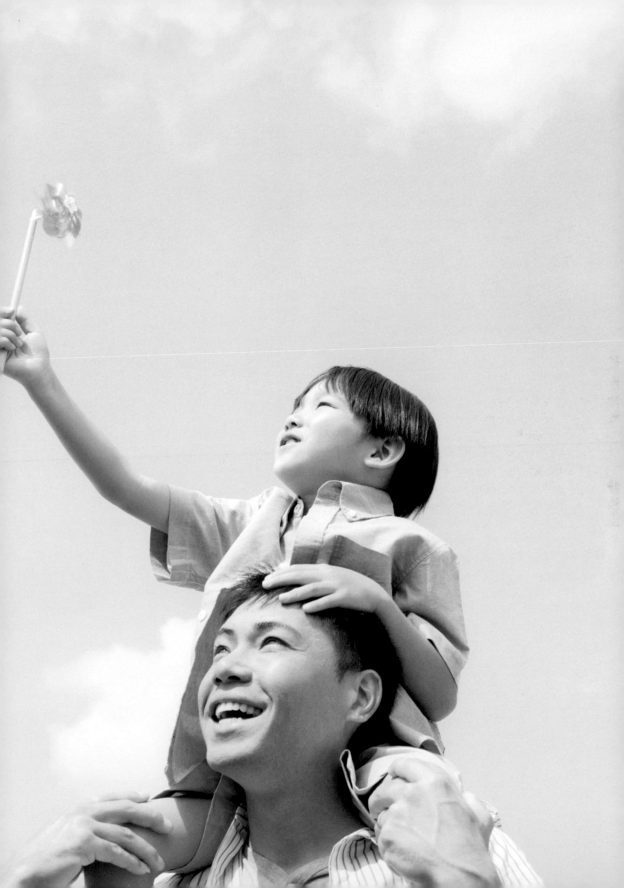

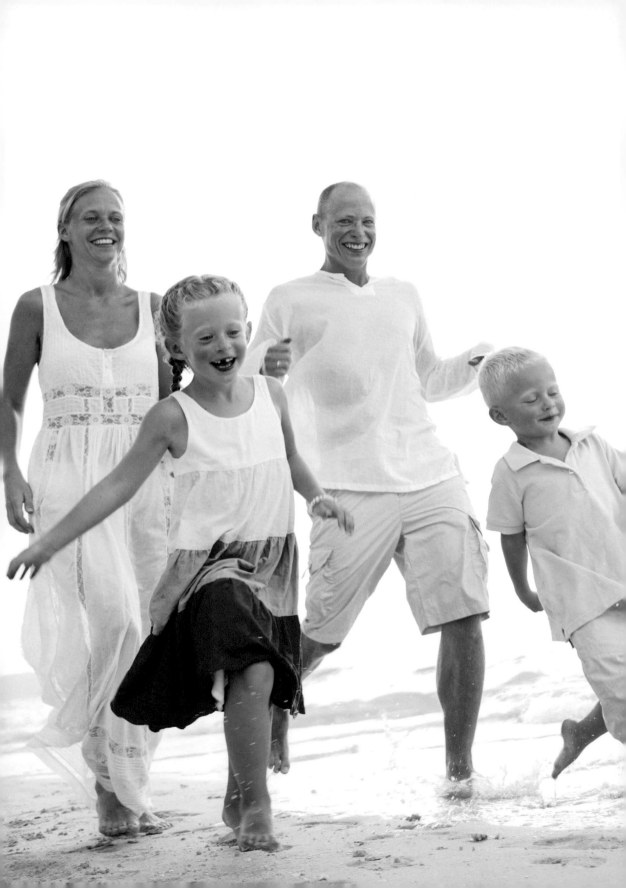

Success stories

Some very impressive cases have been reported over the years.

One of the most amazing is that of a 56-year-old woman from Northern Western Australia. Dorothy's story must settle any doubts about vitamin A's ability to control severe asthma.

When Dorothy first rang, I asked if she would write a detailed account of her illness. She kindly obliged and this is her story:

'I was only five when first diagnosed with asthma. For the following 51 years, asthma was a major factor in my life, deciding what I could and could not do. I had become accustomed to living a life restricted by the disease. My condition continually degenerated over the years, to the point when in February 1998, after being released from a Perth hospital and flying back to my home, I was forced to be removed from the plane in a wheelchair.

I WAS SIMPLY UNABLE TO BREATHE WELL ENOUGH TO WALK.'

When I first read Dorothy's letter, I thought, 'Well, airports these days are huge affairs and it's fairly common for ill or elderly folk to require wheelchairs.' Then I remembered she was referring to a town in Northern Western Australia. How large could that airport be?

In addition, she was returning from a stay in hospital. How effective was her medical treatment?

Dorothy was very ill.

Her letter continued, 'I was unable to make my own bed, sweep my small unit or do my own shopping'. (How frustrating having to rely on others while still so young — well, young in my opinion anyway!)

She listed her treatment program:

• 6 hourly doses of Ventolin-Atrovent via nebuliser

• 2 x daily - 500mg Nuelin

• 2 x daily - 3 puffs Flixotide via spacer

• 40mg Steroids per day

• 2 x daily - 3 puffs Serevent

• Ventolin inhaler

How did she tolerate so much medication? Yet, after all that, she was still unable to make her own bed!

Dorothy's General Practitioner informed her the only weapon left in their fight against asthma was in-house oxygen. 'The mere thought of it terrified me', she wrote, 'I felt I was being sentenced to an indefinite term of sitting and waiting for a heart attack to happen'.

Dorothy added 'Learning of your recovery using vitamins A and E seemed like pure fantasy. I didn't believe for one minute such a simple treatment could work for me. But,' she wrote, 'What did I have to lose?'

She purchased the vitamins and began a daily regime of:

- 60,000 i.u. of vitamin A

- 500 i.u. of vitamin E

- 1000mg of vitamin

Following this, Dorothy wrote, 'I haven't felt better in years. I can walk around the shops, do my own housework and am again learning the art of enjoying life. I no longer require the steroids, the Ventolin/Atrovent nebuliser or the Serevent puffer. Thank you for sharing this wonderful treatment. Breathe easy!' Dorothy rang in June 1998, reporting she was still in excellent health and had spread the vitamin A message as much as she could. She has lost 18 kilograms and walks every evening for half an hour. 'Everyone is astonished!' she said.

As I stated earlier, Dorothy's story dispels any doubts about the ability of vitamin A to work for serious cases.

'I have received hundreds of unsolicited success stories. These are asthmatics that have made the effort to report back. The actual number of recoveries must be much, much higher.

Peter, 14-year-old asthmatic

Peter's parents, who live in Darwin, contacted me in April 1998, to express their excitement at the effect vitamins were having on their son's health.

Peter, aged 14, was very allergic to spear grass, which is prevalent in the Northern Territory. He had been hospitalised every March for the past four years, yet, after commencing vitamins early 1998, in March when spear grass was prolific, Peter suffered no asthma.

When his parents first contacted me he was on Becloforte and Ventolin. His father continued, 'Two years ago when he was 12, he was prescribed 50mg of Prednisolone per day. This caused blurring of vision, disturbances in speech, and he was unable to read the blackboard at school!'

The vitamins began working for Peter within a week.

He continued taking 10,000 i.u. of vitamin A, 200 i.u. of vitamin E and 500mg of vitamin C for about twelve months.

I spoke to his father in July 2000 and he reported Peter no longer suffers asthma and has taken no vitamins for over a year. He also needs no medication.

Mark – An asthmatic for 50 Years

Mark, a psychologist, rang one night from New Zealand. He explained he'd seen my asthma segment on television while holidaying in Australia.

After arriving back in New Zealand, he commenced the vitamins and reported, 'I haven't needed my Ventolin puffer for six weeks.'

'But six weeks isn't very long ' I replied.

'It is for me!' he exclaimed, ' I've had asthma for 50 years and it's been decades since I've gone six weeks without symptoms!'

Mark developed asthma at age five. While he was small he was given adrenaline injections or adrenaline pills to help him through attacks. 'The pills were taken under the tongue and tasted very bitter,' he said. 'They also made my heart pound.'

Between the ages of l5 and 30, he experienced no asthma and he believes his extreme fitness as a rugby union player helped him during that time.

Before beginning the vitamins, he was on Ventolin, Pulmicort and Becotide. Since September 1998, he has been taking:

• 1 dessertspoon Cod Liver Oil = 20,000 i.u. Vitamin A (N.Z.)

• 250 i.u. Vitamin E

• Vitamin C every day

When he was ill, he said his E.P. volume was 240 – 350. When on Ventolin it was 550. Now, without Ventolin, it is still 550.

I spoke to Mark again in August 2000. He told me the vitamins began working within a week, and two years later they were still working beautifully. 'I run and walk each day and I find it absolutely brilliant that I can run up a hill at 59 years of age without using my puffer.'

'I haven't visited the doctor at all this year. In the past I'd be at the surgery every six weeks renewing my medications. It was very expensive. Now I simply buy a bottle of cod liver oil for $11 or $12, and it lasts almost two months. I'm saving a fortune!'

'I also eat lots of fish, green salads and brown rice and I feel this diet helps keep my weight down. I sometime pour extra cod liver oil over my salads. I think being overweight exacerbates asthma.'

All up, Mark is probably taking about 40,000 i.u. of vitamin A.

I was interested to hear him say 1 dessertspoon of New Zealand cod liver oil equals 20,000 i.u. of vitamin A. I was sure Australian oil was not so strong, so when visiting our local chemist I studied the

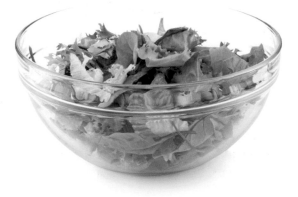

labels on liquid cod liver oil, endeavouring to calculate the quantity of vitamin A in the oil. I couldn't make heads or tails of the measurements, so went home to look up my books. I still couldn't make any sense of it, so rang the chemist and asked her to explain it to me.

She agreed the labels were confusing and told me half a teaspoon of cod liver oil would equal 1,200 i.u. This means 1 dessertspoon would measure almost 5,000 i.u. of vitamin A:

• 1 dessertspoon of cod liver oil in N. Z. = 20,000 i.u. of vitamin A.

• 1 dessertspoon of cod liver oil in Australia = 5,000 i.u. of vitamin A.

I wonder how much vitamin A was in the old Scott's Emulsion we youngsters swallowed in dessert spoons?

Liquid cod liver oil is still strong enough for children, but for adults, Australian cod liver oil in either capsule or liquid form is scarcely worth the bother.

Andrea — No symptoms since 1998

Andrea has experienced a wonderful recovery from her asthma. Since commencing the vitamins in June 1998, she has been free of symptoms.

'I've suffered this illness for 22 years,' she said. 'My brother died at 47 from an asthma attack. In the past I would visit my doctor at least once a month. It's over a year now since I last saw him. It was costing me $100 a month for medication – did you know Serevent is $20 per puffer?'

Andrea's vitamin dose during September and October was:

• 50,000 i.u. of vitamin A

• 500 i.u. of vitamin E

She also eats pawpaw each morning for breakfast. Later she reduced her vitamin A dose to 20,000 i.u. and was still maintaining good health.

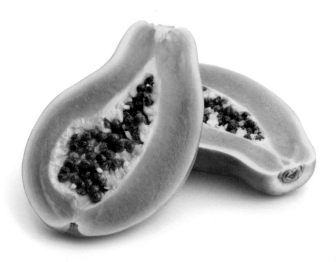

'Asthma is a huge problem in my area,' she said. 'As a teacher I see children sucking on their Ventolin all day.'

Andrea contacted me February 2000 to report she was still asthma- free. 'I'm now down to 15,000 i.u. of A per day and I'm thinking of reducing my vitamin E also.'

'I wouldn't reduce the vitamin E if I were you,' I replied, 'You are now 50, and most experts advise those in their 50s and older to maintain good vitamin E levels. It has a reputation for helping the heart.'

She continued, 'I'm taking no cortisone and very rarely use some Ventolin – nothing else. In the past, I took my nebuliser to work and used it in the common-room.' (That would be embarrassing I would imagine).

'These days, I have more energy than others years younger than myself. But when I mention vitamin A to my work-mates or parents at the school, their eyes glaze over.'

I know what she means. I encounter the same glazing myself. Perhaps others believe 'scare tactics' they've heard regarding vitamin A, and rather than offend us by expressing these negative opinions, they simply glaze over.

The following are copies of a letters I received via the internet

On 23/04/2012 1:44 PM Lisa wrote:

Just wanted to pop by & say hi.

I emailed you a couple of years ago. You may not remember me. We had been through bad health & I developed asthma after being in a mouldy house & I emailed asking about vit A.

I have been going well. After 6 months intensive vit A dosages I didn't take any vit A for well over a year with no asthma. Started getting a little wheezy recently so now again on a maintenance dose. Many of my friends have borrowed your book & having success with it too. Thanks for writing it. I am 35 years old. I always considered myself a healthy fit person until recent years.

A few weeks ago whilst visiting a friend for dinner, they explained that he was advised 3 yrs ago to take vit A by an ambulance driver. Dosage: 1 Tablet on day 1, 2 tablets on day 2, etc until 7 on day 7 ... then decrease them the same way down to 0 again. He did this and hasn't had hay fever again until this year, so he repeated the procedure and again has no hay fever. This prompted my memory of when we lived in Melbourne. A neighbour had a teenage daughter who was rushed to hospital monthly nearly dead from asthma. Just before leaving Melbourne, her mum told me her asthma was totally cured, off all medication due to reading your book "Give Asthma the big A".

Hope you are well.

Lisa

From Facebook

Hi Marian,

Thank you thank you, thank you. I have been taking your advice for only a week & already I have stopped taking Symbicort ... which only barely worked for me.

I am feeling soooo much better & no asthma tightness. I thought I was allergic to almost everything, the constant sneezing, sore & itchy eyes, itchy roof of mouth, constant nasal drip ... just to name a few, are all diminished and improving daily.

I have a question. I am taking Proactive Multi Vitamins which contain 2500 iu Retinyl Palmitate, Natural E 500 iu & Vitamin A 5000iu.

I am 59 years old & have had asthma since I was 45.

My question is: all the vitamin bottles are in iu & you give dosages in mg & units is units "iu" Can you help me I'm taking 3 vitamin A per day & 1 vitamin E but I am unsure of the conversions.

So sorry for being such a pest but I so want to do this correctly,

I hope you have time to reply to me as for the first time in years I am feeling normal....I am overjoyed ... Thank you,

Sincerely Yours, Thanks again!

Sue Ralph

Date: Sat, 20 Feb 2010 12:16:56 +1100
Subject: Re: Give Asthma the Big A

Greetings!

I am a fit forty year old who developed heart issues last year and worked out it was my asthma medication so I have been actively looking for alternatives.

My partner found an old copy of your book when she was at our local shop. I read it with some doubt but took it on anyway.

HOLY SMOKE!!!!!!!!!!!!!!!!!!!!!!!!!!!!!!!!!!

One month later I haven't needed ANY medication and have been able do very intense exercise sessions in heat and/or rain etc with perfect lung function. My heart feels great as it isn't full of asthma medication.

My IBS seems to be 50 to 75% better to boot. Thanks for your wisdom!!

Life is good.

Brad Westfall

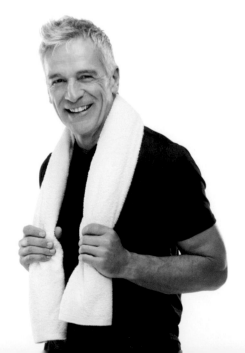

Dear Brad,

Thank you for your absolutely fabulous letter!! I've received many success letters but yours just blew me away! I'm so happy that you have experienced such an amazing reversal of your asthma and that you can enjoy your exercise much more.

Have you always been an asthmatic and which medication do you think was causing your heart problems?

I've joined Facebook in the last week, to try to get the message out a bit more. It surprised me that Americans were talking about the latest FDA Warnings issued on 4 Asthma drugs, namely Advair, Symbicort, Foradil and Serevent. They said these drugs could cause sudden life-threatening worsening of asthma.

On the website msnbc.msn.com there were two other FDA warnings mentioned from 2009 and these were about Xolair (causing heart problems) and Singulair (Psychiatric problems).

The thing that got me is here in Queensland, we have heard of no warnings at all. Actually nothing about asthma has been published in the paper for about 10 years. It's funny because I just mentioned that fact to Jim the day before. Asthma was always in the paper in years gone by.

Do you mind if I ask my son to add your letter to my website www.aforasthma.com.au. I can omit your name if you like.

I'm sure you will continue to enjoy freedom from asthma, as I have myself. Vitamins A and E really are miraculous, aren't they?

Thanks again for your kind words,
Marian Slee.

23rd February, 2010

Hello!

I only developed asthma when I was 32. I am certain that my condition got worse when I was put on Symbicort as I HAD to have it every day after using for a while. When I accidentally ran out I developed very bad headaches till I got a new script. When it happened again I quite easily made the connection. I had also begun to develop heart issues about the same time.

I halved my usage and had constant tightness in my chest as well as discomfort, but couldn't stop totally as I had become dependent on Symbicort. At least when I was on Seritide and ventolin I could wean myself off of it as needed. I was worried about using any medication though as I feared heart attacks at that point. I was sent through tests etc and my heart was deemed very healthy.

That went on for several months and I hoped for something better.

That's when Clare found your 1996 book in Cooranbong.

Fortunately I have a friend who is very well versed in the effect of vitamins and the human body in general. He researched independent findings on the net and your theories were supported elsewhere. Within two days I stopped all medication and haven't needed any medication at all since. I still need to fine-tune my usage of A, E and C, but I'll get there.

I believe it is criminal that such a life-saving and simple "cure" for asthma is so readily available and government bodies etc aren't choosing to stop people from early deaths by being proactive with this obvious great finding.

The whole IBS thing is a HUGE bonus that lends itself to the cortisone/inflammation theory based on the current wisdom that is out there.

Feel free to use my name and information as I too hope lives can be saved!!!!!!!!!!!!!!!!

Thanks again!

Brad Westfall

Date: 01 September 2012 07:14:27 AM

Hi Marian,

I just wanted to write to you and say how thankful I am to have found you! My 4 year old daughter Brooklyn suffers from Asthma and has been hospitalised several times since she was 2 (once in intensive care!).

I hope you don't mind me telling you her story...

Since the age of 2, Brooklyn had been having some health problems including losing weight and bleeding gums. We are located on the NSW Central Coast and were referred to Westmead Children's Hospital where a Dr told us, after numerous tests, Brooklyn has Crohn's Disease. She was one of the youngest in the world to be diagnosed with the disease. We met with an immunologist and gastroenterologist and they agreed that before we try steroids we should try a diet free from preservatives, artificial colours, flavours etc. Well the diet worked wonders! Although, she still had tummy pain, I somehow came across the website www. fedup.com.au and discovered the world of salicylates. As soon as I stopped salicylates her tummy pain stopped! It was amazing! The whole family ate the same way and we have all noticed benefits so have kept it up!

Then the Asthma came. After a few visits to hospital I realised that her asthma was triggered when she gets a cough. She could have a cold and no cough and not develop asthma but as soon as a cough comes, wham! Asthma! It comes on so quick that I end up sleeping with her the same night giving her Ventolin all through the night on the verge of taking her to hospital. As well as sending her crazy the prednisolone reduces her appetite and she is very small already. She lost 1.3kg in a matter of a week!

I was recently talking to a mum at my other daughter's school and she recommended your book so I ordered it straight away. Whilst waiting for it to arrive I started her on Cod Liver Oil tablets (600IU each) of which I was giving her x 3 and 1 x vitamin E tablet (250IU) and half a teaspoon of vit C powder. She developed a cough before I heard about the vitamins recently and had her Ventolin and prednisolone (which by the way makes her Crohn's symptoms worse AND sends her crazy!). The cough went away and I started her on A, E and C and she has since developed another cough with NO ASTHMA! I was sooooo excited! Every cough since she was 2 has resulted in asthma.

I read your book and was very disappointed to get to the end! It was very interesting. I have now got my hands 10000IU of Vit A tablets and give one a day to her. I'm not sure if this is right but she seems fine.

I know it's only early days but I am very excited about your vitamin theory and feel it will really benefit Brooklyn. I will do anything to stop those nasty drugs being pumped into my daughter! (Even though, as you suggest, I keep her Ventolin and prednisolone on hand just in case). Her paediatrician recommended a preventer called Flixotide but it made her constantly crazy and just miserable so we stopped it and just started giving her Ventolin when a cough develops. Now, I will be increasing her dose of vit A when she gets a cough.

Thank you so much for writing your book and spreading the word about Asthma relief. Even though only a few will listen I will be telling everyone I meet about this wonderful theory!

Kind regards,

Shell Naysmith

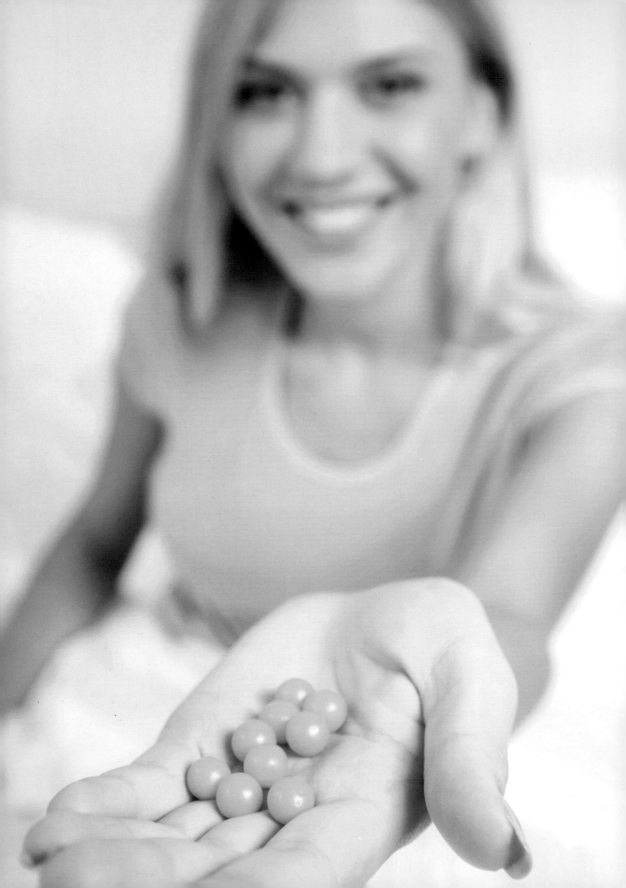

Not all vitamins are equal

In the principal 1999 textbook for Grade 12 Biology, a table of Recommended Daily Allowances of vitamins and minerals stated the RDA for vitamin A was 1 milligram. I'd never seen vitamin A measured in any form except international units (i.u.) so I was convinced it must have been a misprint. However after consulting the book Vitamins and Your Health *by Ann Gildroy, I found that:*

• 1 microgram of vitamin A = 3.3 i.u. of vitamin A, so

• 1 milligram of vitamin A = 3,300 i.u. of vitamin A (1 milligram equals 1,000 micrograms)

Therefore, the Recommended Daily Allowance of 1mg for vitamin A as stated in the textbook is close to correct as this would equal 3,300 i.u. The current RDA is 2,500 units. Anyone reading those measurements in the Biology textbook, however, would assume the Recommended Daily Allowance of vitamin A at 1mg was extremely low, and would not believe it equaled 3,300 i.u.

Many Biology students go on to become doctors. Is it any wonder they appear astonished when a patient states he is taking, say 20,000 i.u. of vitamin A per day.

Vitamin E is also sold in international units. However it's potency is very different from vitamin A:

• 100 i.u. of vitamin E = 67mg

• Fat-soluble vitamins can be very confusing to the uninitiated!

There was another surprising section in the Biology books. In a written exercise, students were asked to ascertain the nutritional status of a girl who went on a three months' diet over the Christmas holidays. During this time she ate nothing but three apples per day. Students were shown a table setting out the vitamin and mineral content of one apple.

I couldn't believe this information! It stated an apple contains seven milligrams of vitamin A plus other vitamins and minerals. We know straight vitamin A is found only in animal products, therefore an apple has absolutely none. Also, as beta-carotene is yellow, I doubt an apple would have much of that either.

One milligram of vitamin A equals 3,300 units, so this apple, supposedly containing seven milligrams, would total 23,100 units. Multiply that by the three apples per day and you have 69,300 i.u. of vitamin A; all from a fruit which would actually have none.

This wouldn't have been so appalling as it could have been a typing error. But in the answers to the exercise, it stated after three months, the girl would be severely deficient in every vitamin and mineral except vitamin A, of which she would have overdosed!

I wonder how many biology students believe they could overdose on vitamin A by eating nothing but three apples per day!

Thank goodness this mistake appeared in the manual, not the official textbook and the school was about to change these books.

In spite of this error, I very much favour measuring vitamin A in milligrams or micrograms. I believe many asthmatics are reluctant to try vitamin A because measuring it in units makes the quantities seem frighteningly high.

Milligrams make more sense, as they are a set measurement, and vitamin A should be sold in that form. Besides, giving a child three milligrams of vitamin A sounds more acceptable than 10,000 i.u. Maybe we should follow the biology textbook and use this measurement more often:

• 3,300 i.u. vitamin A = 1mg vitamin A

• 5,000 i.u. = 1.5mg

• 10,000 i.u = 3mg

• 20,000 i.u = 6mg

• 60,000 i.u. = 18mg

Since 1997 there's been a plentiful supply of 5,000 i.u. vitamin A capsules in the shops. Most Australian vitamin catalogues however, advertise only 2,500 i.u. Fortunately, these companies do stock inexpensive halibut-liver oil capsules of a good strength (4,000 to 5,000 i.u. vitamin A, 10 mcg vitamin D).

Halibut liver oil is excellent if only low doses of vitamin A are needed and because my requirement has dropped, I sometimes take them myself.

Admittedly, it is still not possible to purchase a 10,000 i.u. vitamin A dose and there's no indication this restriction will be lifted. Still, most asthmatics should be able to purchase a 5,000 i.u. capsule which agrees with both their stomachs and budgets.

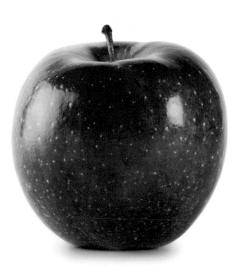

Although my vitamin A requirement is falling, I still can't cease taking them completely because nasal congestion and a dry cough soon develop. I haven't discontinued vitamins until asthma manifests because the nasal congestion is so detrimental to sleep I'm soon forced back on them.

At 58 years of age, with the asthma season in full swing, my daily dosage was only:

• 15,000 to 25,000 i.u. of vitamin A

• 500 i.u. of vitamin E

• half teaspoon calcium acorbate powder (Vitamin C)

Danny, our eldest son is now 47 and seldom needs any vitamins. He appears to have outgrown asthma as he's suffered no attacks since age 21.

When using halibut liver oil, I make a point of taking no more than six capsules per day. This equals 24,000 i.u. vitamin A, and 2,400 i.u.(60 mcg) vitamin D – well below the vitamin D overdose level of 4,000 i.u.(100 mcg). If more vitamin A is needed, straight vitamin A capsules can be added. Because of my age, I sometimes take halibut liver oil capsules as vitamin D should help in the fight against osteoporosis.

When I was 45, a friend exclaimed, 'You're on 60,000 units of vitamin A now! What will you be taking when you're old?'

I must admit, I wondered myself, yet here I am at 71, still needing vitamins A and E but not quite as high a dose as I thought. 60,000 i.u. to 90,000 i.u. seems to keep me healthy. Lady Cilento recommended strong doses of vitamin A in her book *Medical Mother* and I'm glad she did as it gave me the courage to increase this vitamin when needed. However, I've now learned doses don't automatically have to increase with age.

While on the subject of dosages, I must ask for care in reading labels on cod and halibut liver oil capsules. These bottles are usually labeled Cod Liver Oil 275mg or Halibut Liver Oil 145mg. **This is not the measurement of vitamin A in the capsule!** Rotate the bottle until the actual vitamin A and D doses are found. Cod Liver Oil capsules usually contain 580 i.u., or 5,000 i.u. of vitamin A and Halibut Liver Oil about 4,000 i.u. of vitamin A.

I've written to vitamin companies requesting this be changed because it's too easy to confuse the mg measurement of fish oil on the front of the label with the actual quantity of vitamin A and D written on the side of the container. These misleading labels could cause overdosing.

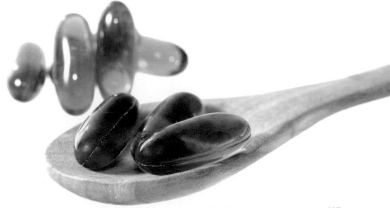

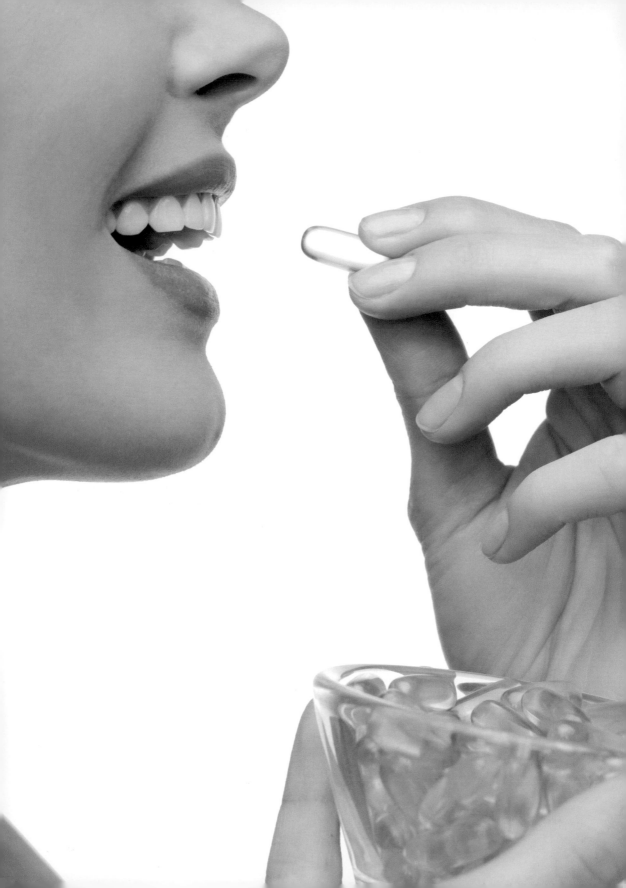

Advantages of vitamins over drugs

Listed below are the tremendous advantages obtained from the use of vitamins (as opposed to drugs) as the principal method of controlling asthma. The most significant of these advantages are:

1. Absence of Side Effects

This is the most wonderful advantage of them all. Unlike sufferers on medication, asthmatics who take the correct dose of A, E and if necessary C, would have no symptoms, no side-effects and could enjoy life to the fullest.

2. Eliminates Fear

Although vitamins take about twenty hours to work, they have a tremendous advantage in that they continue working for at least twelve hours and usually much longer. This eliminates the perpetual worry of parents and patients — that puffers might be mislaid when the asthma sufferer is away from home.

3. Vitamins are Easy and Pleasant to Take

No puffers or machines required. No embarrassment in public. Taking vitamins is more socially acceptable than using a puffer.

The outlay for vitamin treatment depends upon a person's age and the severity of their disease. For children the expense is minimal. If purchased from the distributor, they would consume less than $5 worth of vitamins per month in winter, half that in summer. The costing for adults would range from $5 to $20 per month in winter. Much less in summer. Vitamins are cheaper and fresher if bought in bulk from the distributor.

4. Less Concern Over Long-term Effects

Many asthmatics (and parents of asthmatics) worry about the long- term effects of medication — I did. With vitamin treatment, there is little cause for concern. Any detrimental effect from vitamin overdose is quickly reversed by ceasing or reducing the vitamin. One wonders if adverse reactions to drugs are so easily reversed.

5. Treatment can be Increased Without Fear

During times of severe asthma, vitamin dosages can be significantly increased without fear of overdose. Lady Cilento said adults can safely take 60,000 to 90,000 units of vitamin A for a period of three months. The safety margin for drugs is dramatically lower than for vitamins.

6. Most Asthma Drugs Merely Suppress Symptoms

With vitamins, there are no symptoms. Remember the mother of the 12-year-old girl. She said, 'If they invented a drug as good as this, it would be hailed a wonder drug!'

7. Increased Energy Levels

Provided the correct amount of vitamins is taken, there is a substantial increase in natural (not drug induced) energy.

8. Vitamins Work Quickly

AS A PREVENTATIVE, vitamins A and E work faster than inhaled corticosteroids (Becotide® etc.) which can require up to three weeks to take effect. Despite the popular belief that vitamins require months to be effective, most asthmatics have reported improvement within a few days.

9. Vitamins and Drugs are Compatible

Although I have always tried to avoid medication, many people combine the two with success.

Final recommendations

After reading this book, I'm confident you will feel a new optimism towards your asthma. I'm sure your life-style will be happier and healthier and I hope you will not allow 'scare tactics' to dampen that optimism.

Someone once said 'Fear is Faith in Disaster' and it often seems fear can be stronger than love or life itself. Fear can shrivel us up; reducing our ability to 'have a go' at achieving the good health for which we were designed.

One of the best antidotes to fear is hope. Does anyone, however expert, have the right to tell another, 'There is no hope.' How can they know the future with so much certainty? Don't allow yourself to be frightened off vitamin A.

Keep in mind, ANYTHING is dangerous in overdose, and symptoms of vitamin A overdose are completely reversible within a few days.

THERE IS NOTHING TO FEAR.
Rather than rejecting new ideas, a wise person would agree with my nutritionist who says 'I'm for whatever works.'

I would like to leave you with my personal Winter Health Tips in the hope that you might find them helpful.

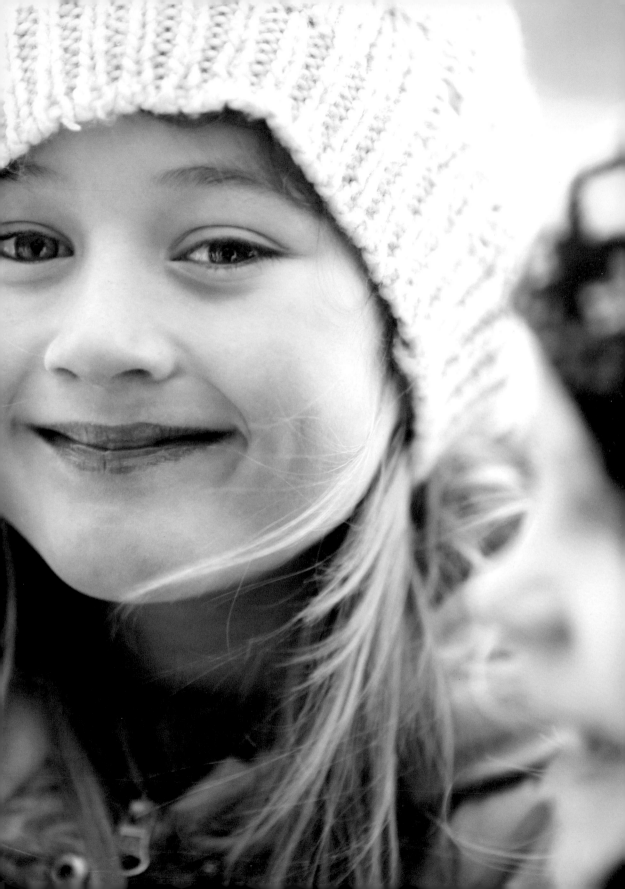

Marian's Winter Health Tips

1. Be aware of fluctuating temperatures.

2. Take vitamins every day in winter, using the minimum amount required to eliminate symptoms.

3. Wear a spencer or woollen vest during cold weather. (Keep the chest and back of neck warm).

4. Invest in a good quilt.

5. Blow-dry hair immediately after shampooing and take a good dose of vitamin C. This helps prevent colds, influenza and ear problems.

6. Avoid taking hot showers immediately before a night out.

7. Wash hands often in winter, as infections are spread by hand contact. Avoid touching face.

8. Keep warm. If the body uses all its energy maintaining normal temperature, it has nothing left to fight infection.

9. Asthmatics should suspect mild asthma if feeling persistently tired. I always increase A and maybe E. (Persistent fatigue, however, is not always asthma-related)

10. If increasing A and E doesn't ease definite asthma symptoms, I treat as a viral infection by increasing vitamin C powder to three teaspoons per day for five days. Use much smaller doses for children.

11. Vitamin E must not be increased quickly if you suffer high blood pressure.

12. Do not take iron tablets and vitamin E at the same time as iron can cancel out vitamin E. (from The Vitamin Conspiracy).

13. I usually commence vitamins in late February or early March.

14. Temperatures can drop suddenly around this time.

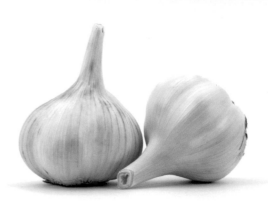

15. If overcome by a cold or influenza, don't assume vitamins have failed and give up. This is the time to increase vitamin intake if asthma is to be avoided.

16. Always include plenty of vitamin A rich foods in your diet and use garlic occasionally in cooking. Garlic has a reputation for being beneficial in asthma — not so for romance!

17. In case of emergencies, make sure asthma medications are on hand and up to date.

18. Asthma should never be taken lightly. Severe asthmatics should organise a crisis plan with a doctor. A Peak Flow Meter is advisable.

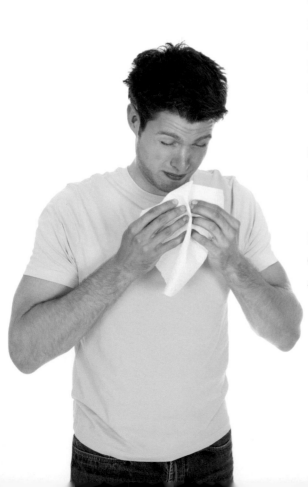

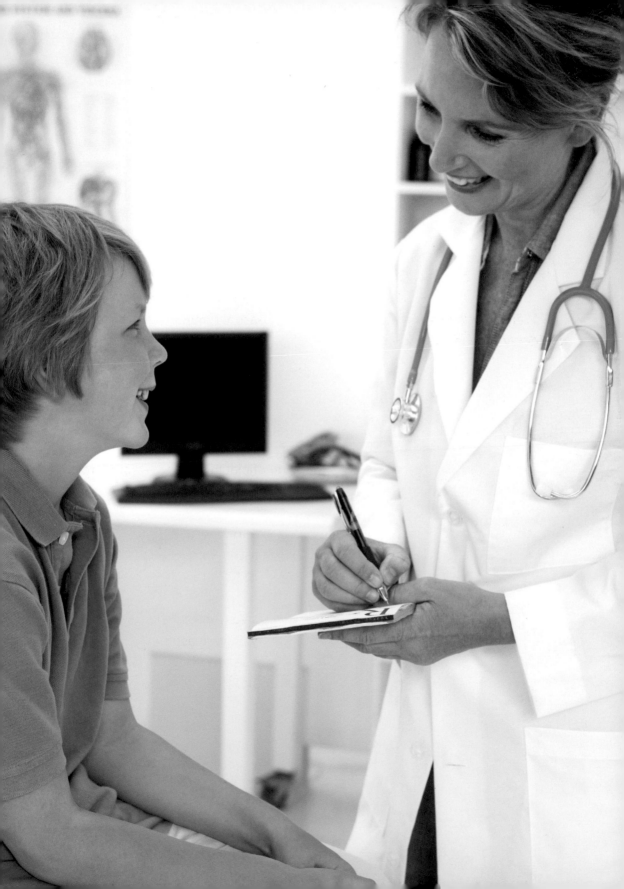

No one can know the future. For the rest of our lives, these vitamins may be all that I and others on this programme, will require.

If, while rearing a large family, I had been continually suffering asthma symptoms or side-effects from drugs, I would have found life impossible, so I was virtually forced to find a cure for my malaise. You can understand then why I am so excited about this vitamin treatment.

I feel sure, that we who have known success with vitamins, will always be grateful for QUALITY OF LIFE, and isn't that one of the most important things of all?

I can't imagine any medication capable of controlling asthma, hayfever and nasal problems for a period of thirty-four years. This simple treatment is indeed miraculous.

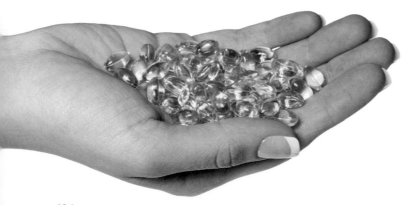

Bibliography

This is not the place for a definitive bibliography on asthma. The following is simply a list of books which helped me.

Adams, R. and Murray, F. *Improving Your Health With Vitamin A* (U.S.A.: Larchmont Books, 1978)

Alexander, P. *It Could be Allergy and It Can be Cured* (Australia: Ethicare Pty.Ltd., 2000)

Antia, F.P. *Clinical Dietetics and Nutrition* (Bombay: Oxford University Press, 1989)

Atkins, R.C. *Dr Atkins' Nutrition Breakthrough* (New York: William Morrow and Co. Inc., 1981)

Bingham, S. *Dictionary of Nutrition* (London: Barrie & Jenkins, 1977)

Cilento, P. Lady *Medical Mother* (Australia: *The Courier Mail* Publication, 1982)

Cilento, P. Lady *Vitamin and Mineral Deficiencies* (Australia: Pitman Publishing Pty. Ltd., 1983)

Colgan, M. *Your Personal Vitamin Profile* (Great Britain: Blond & Briggs, 1984)

Davis, D. *Are You Poisoning Your Family?* (Australia: Lamont Publishing, 1991)

Fried, J.J. *The Vitamin Conspiracy* (USA: Clarke Irwin & Co., 1975)

Gerras, C *The Complete Book of Vitamins* (USA: Rodale Press, Emmaus, PA, 1977)

Gildroy, A. *Vitamins and Your Health* (Great Britain: Unwin Paperbacks, 1983)

Gregg, I. *Asthma — Its Management in General Practice* (Australia: Update Publications, 1985)

Hayes, W.J. Jr. *Toxicology of Pesticides* (Baltimore: the Williams and Wilkins Company, 1975)

Lankford, T.R. and Steward, P.J. *Foundations of Normal and Therapeutic Nutrition* (New York: Wiley, 1986)

Meillon, R. and Reading, C. *Relatively Speaking* (Sydney: Fontana Australia, 1985)

Morley, J. *Beta-Adrenoceptors in Asthma* (London: Academic, 1984)

Newbold, H.L. *Vitamin C Against Cancer* (U.S.A.: Stein & Day, 1979)

Snyder, W., Kennedy, E., and Aubusson P., *Biology — The Spectrum of Life* (Melbourne: Oxford University Press,1990)

Wills, E.D. *Biochemical Basis of Medicine* (Bristol: Wright, 1985)

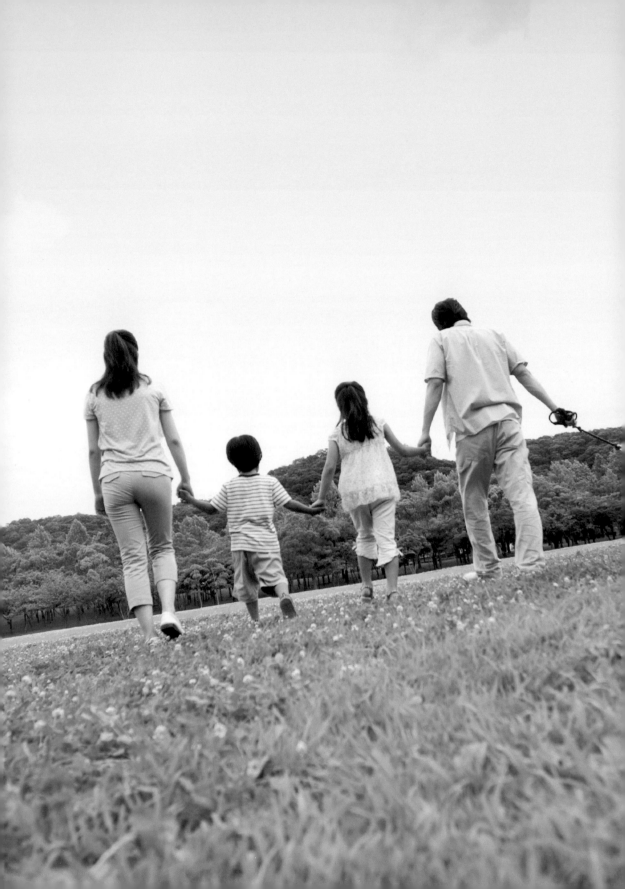

Thank you for reading my book.
I hope you have enjoyed it and I'm sure
you will find it helpful in your fight
against asthma.

When we are in good health,
life's joys are enhanced and the
difficulties are easier to handle.

This is my wish for you then – vibrant good health!

Best wishes - Marian Shepherd Slee

www.aforasthma.com.au

Index

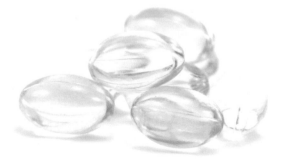